I BEAT CANCER

I BEAT CANCER

Dan Cornish

I BEAT CANCER

ISBN: 978-1-7322232-5-7
eBook ISBN: 978-1-7322232-4-0

Printed in the United States of America
10 9 8 7 6 5 4 3 2 1
First Edition

"The human body and mind are tremendous forces that are continually amazing scientists and society. Therefore, we have no choice but to keep an open mind as to what the human being can achieve." - Evelyn Glennie

To my Dad, who's beating cancer as I did

CONTENTS

INTRODUCTION

The motivation for this book was reading a huge variety of books and medical papers while I was trying to defeat prostate cancer and being frustrated by the sheer daily difficulty and cost not only of following the treatments in all these vastly divergent books for my own cancer. My own highly technical background as an engineer and medical science and bio-hacking freak reading up on cancer had given me excellent ideas on how to approach it and I devised a three-pronged approach not only to keep the cancer at bay but quickly diminish and then finally eliminate it entirely. For me the term remission did not exist - removal was a more apt term or as you will see from a newer understanding of cancer, a return to complete good health and best of all with no invasive procedures in the mix. Hard to believe ? Read on. I promise to explain the methodology well.

So why would you read this book ? Others have written books on prostate cancer, how to survive cancer and so on. Well, no-one has written a book on how you can both survive prostate cancer, keep it at bay, preserve your Mojo and look like a man doing it! And how many books will tell you how to treat and cage your prostate cancer for good ? Let's admit it - no such book has been written.

Yet when you read this book you will come to understand like me, how ridiculously easy and less fortuitous this is, requires little discipline and wonder why you need to go through all those unnecessary treatments that make you leave you feeling violated, emasculated and at the end of it all with a big bill to pay off. Talk about giving away a man's dignity. I should know about it just as any survivor of prostate cancer now and in the past.

During the pandemic, many would-be patients put off necessary medical procedures to avoid the risk of COVID. So now there's a backlog of patients in line for surgeries and other procedures. That includes cancer patients at different stages. Once you read this book, you'll see how you can keep going regardless of the current situation. The COVID situation with the lockdowns never had an effect on me. I am totally independent of any problems related to future lockdowns or lurking coronaviruses. That makes me very, very independent of whatever the situation may be.

On the way, you will learn a lot about the more interesting parts of the cancer you can work on and how you can quickly nurse yourself back to health using the three-pronged approach I share in this book. To you my fellow reader, live long and prosper!

Dan Cornish.

The Cheapskate's guide to beating cancer

Here's my story in a nutshell. I was stricken with prostate cancer in the spring of 2017. I didn't know it was growing and by the time I found it was three years too late. Thank God, it was a slow growing cancer, which is what prostate cancer is supposed to be. It could be in your body for a decade or two and if you didn't get your prostate checked regularly, sometimes you might never know till it was already too late.

I was running a small business at the time. While looking at ways to grow the business, I had issues that my primary doctor first identified as BPH (benign prostate hyperplasia). He suggested Cipro(flaxen) and Kegels to control the urge to urinate many times at night. I think you know the feeling well, my fellow prostate cancer sufferers and survivors! Little did he know that the germ of a tumor was already growing in my prostate. By the time it was discovered it would be Stage 2. But maybe it didn't make a difference in the long run what stage it was. Cancer is cancer, after all, it grows, and does not relent.

I figured having been well educated in years to the synergy

between good food and good healthcare and a form of self-treatment I had practiced through the years that I would attempt to try something myself using the knowledge I had gained. That way, I would avoid burning a hole in my pocket as well as possibly my prostate in due course. And this I hoped to do with not a little amount of optimism. You see, I had been preparing for the better part of decade for just this thing. When it struck, I rolled into action.

My story

My own exposure to the wide world of prostate cancer started years after I had already been diagnosed with BPH or benign prostate hyperplasia by my family doctor. It started with 7-8 trips to the toilet at night, little sleep, irritability, lack of energy mostly from lack of sleep. For the next three years, I was prescribed Cipro by my doctor and told to perform pelvic exercises like Kegels to control my urge to urinate by improving my bladder muscles. I stuck to the gym instead putting in about at least two sessions a week at 30 minutes each, which works to about 10 minutes a day with a good measure of squats thrown in, hoping it would magically "relieve" my bladder pressure.

For three years, I had not known enough to go to a urologist and my PSA level had kept increasing steadily from 2.2 to 4.5 and then higher to 6.1 when I was finally diagnosed with the tumor. My family doctor did not expect a cancer to manifest at such an early age of 47 and neither did I. And so the treatments for BPH continued which consisted of more Cipro and more Kegels til in my third year, I got a new family physician as the old one moved practice and my PSA was now up to 6.1. This physician referred me to an urologist at a hospital in downtown Dallas and one fine Monday morning I showed up at the offices of a wise and wizened old physician, in his late 60s and submitted myself to a rectal exam after being told that PSA levels of that high number were unusual for some especially if one was below 50.

The doctor found a hardened mass with the DRE and referred me to the lab on the first floor of the hospital where I went through my very first(and hopefully last) MRI. A week later I was back in his office, this time with my wife who was by this time growing more concerned at the possibility of what was coming. The doctor told me that he recommended a biopsy, the reason being the tumor was almost 10 mm or 1 cm long and with such a high PSA, a biopsy would be needed to check if the mass was tumorous. He hinted that in the not so recent past, in his 60s, he had a tumor that was only 4 mm that had to be treated with chemotherapy and surgically incised and he hinted that he expected something of that sort on the lines of treatment I would have to undergo once. The high PSA, and more importantly the rate of PSA increase over the years in a relatively short period and the size of the growth that had gone unnoticed for three years made him only more sure of what was coming.

I knew what was coming - the chemotherapy drugs or surgical incision or whatever cornucopia of oncological treatment was going to be scheduled. I said I would opt instead for active surveillance. The doctor at this point had me sign a form saying that I absolved him of any decision in my prostate cancer treatment since I had personally decided not to undergo any further treatment till further notice. With that I left and launched my own treatment schedule from day one that led to my own cure from prostate cancer and continuing success in staying that way. The pages that follow will detail what not only what I did but what you can do yourself to get on the road to recovery without putting yourself through a cornucopia of treatment by which you are confused or if you have started said path, how to help yourself recover faster and completely and if you are simply following a period of active surveillance, how you can without sleepless nights fearing the future, put yourself on the road to recovery starting right now.

Some of these things you may have read in other books but some will be new to you. I suggest you try the three-pronged approach in this book and you will start to see results in little as a few months starting with a reduced PSA, lower incidence of unwanted trips to the toilet, a more active lifestyle, no discomfort and keeping your Mojo and your manliness intact. To you dear reader I wish you all the best. If I can do it so can you. All you have to lose is the discomfort and the pain and in its place you will gain new life, increased energy, continued good health and little or no recurrence of the initial cancer, with chances of survivability vastly improved and longevity of life intact.

The three pronged strategy will be easy to follow and will require little change in your lifestyle. You will welcome these changes especially when you realize that they are not very different from your daily routine, with minor workable additions to it. The whole process is designed to be as less intrusive as possible. And for me as a typically lazy person who puts in the least effort and gets the most results, it had to be that way to be viable for me for the long term. In other words as easy as pie which was exactly how it eventually turned out to be.

Identifying the root cause first

First things first, I could continue in my healthy but slightly suspicious lifestyle as I did before the cancer. You see I was a fitness buff. My daily aim in terms of food intake was to take 1.6 grams of protein per kilogram of body weight. This magic formula was arrived at after years of trial and error when I was at the cusp of my second half of my 100-year lifetime achievement goal. This magic formula also corresponded to protein intake advice from a set of experts who also arrived at 1.6 grams per kg of body weight.

Now I had a problem with eggs beforehand - I could not eat more than one a day without significant constipation. That should have been a warning sign. Thanks to my otherwise very healthy lifestyle, I zeroed into the possibility of eggs and a certain fried chicken sandwich I used to consume on a daily basis to supply an additional fifteen grams of protein. At 205 pounds, I needed to consume 140 grams of protein and the eggs and the fried chicken sandwich was getting me there. No, I was not taking 250 grams a day like some bodybuilders do. So I did some simple research and found that the two things I had added to my diet were possibly the greatest risk factors for cancer, according tor the experts. So the day after my rectal exam, I eliminated both the eggs and fried chicken sandwich. So much for following Arnold the Oak. As I show later, I did not eliminate eggs completely after I had got the cancer in remission. I just followed the cancer experts' recommendations on eggs instead. Neither did I feel the need to entirely eliminate meat from my diet. Curious ? Read on.

Cancer is a metabolic disease

Otto Heinrich Warburg, a German physiologist, medical doctor, and 1931 Nobel laureate in Medicine hypothesized that cancer growth is caused by tumor cells generating energy (as, e.g., adenosine triphosphate/ATP) mainly by anaerobic breakdown of glucose (known as fermentation, or anaerobic "respiration" / respiration without oxygen). This is in contrast to healthy cells, which mainly generate energy from oxidative breakdown of pyruvate.

Pyruvate is an end product of glycolysis(the breakdown of glucose and sugars by enzymes, releasing energy and pyruvic acid) and is oxidized within the mitochondria (the cell's energy factory). Hence, according to Warburg, cancer should be interpreted as a mitochondrial dysfunction. When Warburg served as an officer in the German army, Albert Einstein, who had been a friend of Warburg's physicist father Emil, wrote to

Warburg asking him to leave the army and return to academia, since it would be a tragedy for the world to lose his talents. In total, he was nominated for the Nobel award 47 times over the course of his career. Einstein's work in physics had a great influence on Warburg's biochemical research.

In 1944, Warburg was nominated for a second Nobel Prize in Physiology by Albert Szent-Györgyi, for his work on nicotinamide, the mechanism and enzymes involved in fermentation, and the discovery of flavin (in yellow enzymes).

Several scientists who worked in Warburg's lab, including Sir Hans Adolf Krebs, went on to win the Nobel Prize in future years. Krebs is credited with the identification of the citric acid cycle (or Krebs cycle).

Warburg himself stated "Cancer, above all other diseases, has countless secondary causes. But, even for cancer, there is only ONE PRIME CAUSE. Summarized in a few words, the prime cause of cancer is the replacement of the respiration of oxygen in normal body cells by a fermentation of sugar."

Today Otto Warburg has been proven right. The implications for oncology are tremendous as this turns current accepted theories of cancer on its head.

Hundreds of billions of dollars spent in the so-called "war on cancer" have been wasted in pursuit of a fleeting permanent cure for a cause not properly understood in the first place. The only real benefit of all those billions spent is the development of complex new tools to scan and find tumors, at best a side effect for a cancer patient whose primary aim is just to stay alive.

In 2012, following Otto's work, Thomas N. Seyfried, PhD published a book called Cancer as a Metabolic Disease. Dr. Seyfried has resurrected Otto Warburg's theory of cancer causation and confirmed it. For a few oncologists, albeit a few the light has finally turned on. One oncologist has called it the most significant finding in his 50 years of cancer treatment and study.

What came first - the Chicken or the egg ?

The mainstream theory is that cancer is caused by genetic mutations – damage to the DNA. Warburg's theory was that the mitochondria is damaged first, before the DNA is severely damaged. DNA and mitochondria are both damaged by: carcinogenic hydrocarbons, viruses, radiation (X-rays, ionizing & UV), build up of reactive oxygen species (ROS) and inflammation.

The damaged cells begin to divide uncontrollably; they live virtually forever instead of dying off naturally (apoptosis). They develop their own network of blood vessels (angiogenesis).

However DNA is damaged all the time, without turning a cell cancerous, because in healthy DNA there are certain genes that repair the DNA strand when it's damaged, and other genes that tell the cell it's time to die after it's been around for a while.

The DNA theory is mistaken, and as a result almost no progress has been made in cancer treatment. A scientist today cannot get a grant to conduct research in the first place if the proposed project isn't an offshoot of the DNA theory.

Remember, a few gene mutations do not cause cancer. Many people who have them don't get cancer. The reason for this is the presence of other genes that repair DNA. Yes those are real. If those reparative genes were not present, in today's toxic environment, virtually EVERYONE would get cancer.

Respiration is the process by which a healthy cell generates energy. Fermentation is a fallback process for generating energy that the mitochondria will use only when they're damaged and unable to perform respiration or when there's a temporary lack of oxygen, a key component in the normal respiration process.

Cancer cells are different: They make energy by fermentation, not respiration. In this process, the mitochondria turn glucose i.e. sugar (mainly from carbohydrates) into small quantities of energy.

Carbohydrates and especially sugar are the foods cancer needs to feed on. Cancer cells cannot ferment fats. Fermentation is inefficient. It doesn't produce nearly as much energy and creates toxic byproducts – lactic acid and ammonia.

Cancer cells are different not because their DNA is damaged but because they use fermentation even when plenty of oxygen is around. That's what Dr. Seyfried and Warburg mean when they say that cancer is a metabolic disease rather than a genetic disease.

If you deny cancer cells glucose, it is impossible for them to stay alive. Those that do survive will likely be eliminated by your immune system.

So the most likely explanation is that most of the damage to DNA comes after the damage to mitochondria, when the cell is sick and the fermentation process is producing massive amounts of toxic fermentation byproducts.

If you have cancer it becomes important to limit all sugar, in any form, as well as refined carbohydrates like flour and other high-glycemic foods like potatoes or rice. You then starve cancer cells of their food.

The urgent question for you is - do you really want to wait till Otto Warburg is eventually proven right, in maybe another 100 years ? Will you even be around for that by the time most oncologists realize that he was indeed right ?

Bring in the cavalry

Imagine you are face to face with a bully walking alone at night in a dark alley. You try your best to stand your ground but this bully is 7 feet tall, muscular and looks like he could beat the pants out of two of you at the same time. You raise yourself up to full height, stand your ground and warn the bully - "You better not make a move or you're going to regret it!"

The bully simply smiles and calls your bluff grinning fiendishly "Oh yeah, you and what army ?"

Now imagine the 7 foot tall bully is the cancer inside, ravaging your body, it seems to grow without limit day by day fiendishly taking over new territory. The cancer is smug till you realize that you have a small army in your reach you could use to actually beat the bully. And where is the cavalry so as to speak? They are right there in your body, part of your alimentary system, in your gut. The weight of this cavalry is typically 3 lbs and consists of trillions of good bacteria (along with bad). Some of these bacteria are lactobacillus acidophilus, lactobacillus reuteri, lactobacillus rhaminosus and if you seed your gut well, you can have trillions of different probiotic organisms at any time keeping you gut happy, your mind very happy, less depressed and fighting fit, ready to take on most of your enemies within.

Probiotics are a large family of foods - you can take probiotic supplements - they come in high quality and cheap at 60 billion beneficial bacteria per capsule once a day, add some kimchi (Korean fermented cabbage) you'd get these days event at Walmart(probably the only reason I buy food from Walmart these days rather than from a farmer's market). You could try kefir - you could make it yourself from coconut water or milk using different grains for each - called water kefir or milk kefir grains, take yoghurt at least if you dont take probiotics. But kefir is always better than yoghurt and store brought kefir still contains 16 different strains of bacteria you won't find in home made yoghurt and definitely not in store yoghurt. Some of these strains are lactobacillus reuteri, lactobacillus acidophillus and lactobacillus gondarii.

Another thing, when you increase more probiotics in your diet whether through kefir from the Caucasus, Korean kimchi, German sauerkraut or otherwise, you will see small changes (not just a decrease in your beer belly), to a increased hankering within for healthier foods. This shift will happen well before you know it as you start refusing the ground meat burgers and go for better cuts of grass-fed meat or start liking fish and eating your probiotics. All this is good and will help you in defeating the enemy.

A funny thing is happening in the world of cancer treatment. It's subtle. People who don't read about cancer on a regular basis may not notice it. But ever so slowly, the pendulum on treatment is swinging back around from the mania for invasive drugs and procedures to a focus on the immune system.

Instead of coming up with weapons to directly kill cancer cells, immunotherapy helps the immune system do the killing. It seeks to arm the body's immune system with tools needed to fight specific aspects of cancer. There are new breakthroughs in immune therapy. And in contrast to the most powerful high-tech and chemical medical creations the world has ever seen, this pivots toward the tiniest, most basic of all healing organisms: your gut bacteria.

One immunotherapy treatment uses drugs called immune checkpoint inhibitors, which are able to block proteins produced by cancer cells that protect them against immune cells. But not all types of cancer respond to treatments using immune checkpoint inhibitors. Side effects from these drugs can also be severe. So it's fascinating and downright promising that a new study from Nature Communications documents the discovery of a link between gut bacteria and anti-tumor immunity. Building on this research, scientists should be able to pinpoint people most likely to benefit from cancer treatment through immune checkpoint inhibitors. Anti-tumor immunity no longer wishful thinking It all starts with the way gut bacteria interact with the immune system to fight cancer. In the study, multiple strains of gut bacteria were identified as helping to slow the growth of melanoma in mice.

The researchers were part of a large international team that included collaboration with three hospitals. They used mice that lack something called the RING finger protein 5 (RNF5), which helps cells remove rogue proteins. The research revealed that among the RNF5-deficient mice, those with healthy immune systems and intact gut microbe populations were able to stop melanoma – a deadly, highly aggressive cancer. Incredibly, if those same RNF5-lacking mice were housed with mice that did not lack the protein, the animals lost their ability to fight off the melanoma tumors. The same thing happened if the RNF5-lacking mice were treated with antibiotics. Both examples show the enormous role microbes play when it comes to antitumor immune defenses, and how susceptible they are to environment. The investigators even highlighted a signaling pathway known as unfolded protein response (UPR) as the link between the gut bacteria and the antitumor fighting ability of the immune system. UPR appears to be a solid marker for selecting patients with melanoma who are more likely to benefit from immune checkpoint therapy.

According to senior study author Ze'ev Ronai, a professor at Sanford Burnham Prebys in La Jolla, California, the results of the study pinpoint a group of bacterial strains "that could turn on antitumor immunity and biomarkers that could be used to stratify people with melanoma for treatment with select checkpoint inhibitors." They concluded the components of the immune system in the gut, plus the reduction in UPR in both immune and gut cells, played a role in activating the immune cells. The investigators took the research one step further and identified 11 strains of bacteria in the RNF5-lacking mice. When they transplanted those strains to mice with no gut bacteria, an entire antitumor response was triggered and tumor growth decreased.

So, what does this mean for you ? If you're interested in immunotherapy, at the very least start the conversation with your own gut microbiome first. This gives you a further reason to eat a diet that supports a healthy gut. New findings presented at the 2019 Annual Meeting for the American Association for Cancer Research support the idea. Researchers looked at patients just starting treatment and determined that a high-fiber diet, that supplies pre-biotics, which leads to more diverse intestinal bacteria, is linked to a stronger response to Anti-PD-1, an immunotherapy that helps the immune system recognize cancer cells as dangerous.

In this study, researchers collected fecal samples from over 100 people receiving treatment for melanoma and compared tests for gut bacteria to a survey each participant completed about their diets. Their findings show a high-fiber diet, abundant in vegetables, fruits, and whole grains, was associated with the types of bacteria previously linked to better response to anti-PD-1 therapy.

Separately, the researchers looked at a group of almost 50 patients who supplied information on diet and gut microbiome and determined those on a high-fiber diet were about five times more likely to respond favorably to anti-PD-1 treatment than those who ate a low-fiber diet. Better food = Better outcomes, always Researchers plan to run tests on the "antitumor powers" of those antitumor molecules produced by the gut bacteria of the mice that fought cancer to figure out which probiotics might increase the effectiveness of those same molecules in people with melanoma. But at the end of the day, the truth is simple. A high-fiber diet, heavy on a variety of plant-based foods, leads to more diversity in your gut flora, and more diversity strengthens your immune system, and that gives you better outcomes in the prevention and treatment of cancer.

Centenarians in Japan prove the importance of bacteria

Data from a group of centenarians whose average age was 107 revealed gut microbiota that include Odoribacteraceae, which reliably produces a bile acid called isoallo-lithocholic acid, are important to preventing illness. A strong balance of beneficial gut microbiota may also help lower chronic inflammation, which is associated with atherosclerosis, cardiovascular disease, frailty and early death.

Eating probiotic fermented foods to seed your gut microbiome and prebiotic foods rich in insoluble fiber to nourish the beneficial bacteria is an important strategy to benefit your health and wellness. More ways to optimize your gut health are to eliminate sugar, implement a cyclical ketogenic diet and use antibiotics sparingly. Fasting is another strategy that helps support autophagy, boost growth hormone and burn calories.

Researchers from Keio University School of Medicine in Tokyo, Japan, recently released data after studying the gut microbiome of centenarians living in Japan. What they discovered was a unique bacterium that produced a type of bile acid, which seemed to be common to most of the study participants.

While some of the participants exhibited low levels of inflammation, ScienceAlert reports the researchers wrote that "the majority of centenarians were free of chronic diseases such as obesity, diabetes, hypertension (high blood pressure), and cancer."

So if you are after the long life like the Japanese, feed those bacteria!

You don't have to lose your mojo

Contrary to what men think of the dreaded prostate cancer, you don't have to lose your Mojo, feel emasculated or lose your dignity as a man in the process of beating prostate cancer. I gave up nothing and if anything at the end of my prostate cancer experience, I gained in terms of better food, better meat and no longer had any problem down there, if you know what I mean. Starting at a peak of high enuresis, or going to the bathroom 6-8 times a night at the ripe old age of 47, I now drink a glass of water or two before bed and don't wake up till it is time in the morning to wake up. And I'm not making this up. You will see in the pages of this book how it all worked out, with a few tweaks in diet, with a revolutionary new cancer fighting protocol, without completely giving up red meat and even without worrying about waking up in the night if I felt thirsty and needed a drink before bed.

I did not go through any surgery, none at all, no more biopsies, no radial prostatectomy, no chemo and no unwanted drugs. I even dropped Cipro and nursed myself back to full health simply by starting with an inventory of all the foods and drugs I was taking. First off I was always taking vitamin D3 and a multivitamin. Here in the West, most people are deficient in Vitamin D, especially during the winter months. Vitamin D has been implicated in 30% of biochemical processes in the body and it is the sunshine vitamin though there is sometimes little sunshine especially in the winter and your body rarely makes enough of it. So first you need to take inventory. What are you eating and drinking ? Yes, drinking too. Do you know that drinking fruit juice can add tens of pounds to your weight even keeping every other food the same in your diet ? Better to eat the fruit, get the fiber than drink fruit juice and load up with sugar. Cancer LOVES sugar.

Your Mojo gets better than before, you will be vigorous, healthy and happy. Isn't that what every man wants as he grows older? Sadly most do not realize that food is not only needed for sustenance but is also a form of medicine. But today there is a subtle shift in diet as more people eschew carbonated drinks, soda and processed foods. Its only the beginning of a new revolution against cancer and other diseases.

Cancer fighting properties of anti-cancer foods

Turmeric is a potent anti-cancer spice commonly used in Indian cuisine. You can add a pinch of turmeric - and when I mean a pinch, I mean less than 1/4 teaspoon along with paprika to any meat you cook for an extra zing. Don't add too much or it will zing your tongue. The turmeric plant is now recognized for its anti-tumor properties in the West and several higher potency curcumin supplements are available if you don't want to add this to your own food. Recipes incorporating turmeric are available at the end of this book.

Several other cancer fighting ingredients can be found in many sources - like laetrile tea, essiac tea, etc. While I never tried these personally, you might find that these help also in controlling tumor growth. The reason I did not go after such exotic items is that I wanted to see how far I could go with everyday items available at your grocery store and on a budget. I was pretty sure that these items would not necessarily help treat cancer but simply arrest growth. Eventually to treat cancer you need some form of medicine, whether that's chemo or some other drug or remedy. This is an inescapable fact unless you've had surgery already to remove any existing tumor and have then gone the whole nine yards juicing daily, something I did not want to do for the rest of my life. While you can slow down cancers with the above foods or drinks, if you are not careful, it will eventually return as many have found to their detriment. You need to EXCISE the source of radiating cancer in your body with REAL medicine, if not expensive surgery that may be needed from time to time.

All cancer fighting fruits and vegetables The recommended dose is 5-7 servings of fruits and vegetables. Let me confess that I hardly got 1-2 servings a day in the midst of my work and that is counting fruits AND vegetables. Consumption of these cancer fighting fruits and vegetables will help but it is not sufficient by itself. Still pop in as much as you can into your mouth whenever you can and within reach. It makes it that much easier in your fight.

Know what you eat

"Food is medicine" - Paracelsus

The benefits of cooking your own food are enormous. For one, you know what's going into that meal. You know what you use to cook that meal. You know whether you have fried some of it or all of it. And trust me, when you have prostate cancer or ANY cancer you want to stay off fried foods. COMPLETELY. That means fried chicken and fish, the latter which you can substitute with a safer baked version of the same meal. There are recipes in a separate chapter at the end of this book for some really tasty meals that take less than a half hour to prepare. You can cook and refrigerate for a few days these tasty meals and your body will thank you for cooking for it!

Food you can incorporate - cold water fish, plenty of fresh

fruits - all kinds of berries, beans. You don't have to be legalistic about it. You don't have to go organic but do exercise caution if you have a sweet tooth for strawberries. Even though apples are in the dirty dozen, you don't need to go organic as long as you wash them well. An apple a day does keep the doctor away because the pectin goes a long way. Modified citrus pectin is also available cheaply, that's from the white stringy stuff on the inside of an orange that one usually throws away for the fruity stuff inside.

When choosing fish, go for cold water fish when possible - salmon, sardines, etc are best value for the money. Avoid farmed fish especially farmed salmon. You will find that farmed salmon not only is bad for you but also costs more than wild salmon you can pick by the pound, skinless even at places like the frozen food isle at your grocery store. Your aim is to not let go of red meat completely if you like red meat but simply substitute more fish. You can eat cold water fish twice a day for 5 days a week with no issues except a better brain and lots of good omega-3 and to balance out your omega 3 to omega 6 ratio, a huge plus in your cancer fight. Just stick to wild not farmed. You can still eat grass-fed meat 2-3 meals a week and your body will handle it just fine, unless you are into ground meat hamburgers. Go for fresh cuts of meat instead, not the ground mechanically separated meat you find in burger patties. Your body will thank you for it.

Try some pomegranate juice, eat stock on more pumpkin seeds from your local farmers market, sprouts or elsewhere. And don't go too crazy on organics though I would recommend trying to get grass-fed beef rather than the usual corn fed variety. While grass fed meat tastes more earthy there is a perceptible difference from corn fed meat. Your stomach will also feel different as you make the shift. Trust me, try out and you'll see the vast difference in the way your stomach "feels".

Add more tomatoes, add more medicinal mushroom like the 14-mushroom extract from Swanson vitamins to improve immunity, eat more nuts including Brazil nuts, nothing exotic, pick up the mixed fruits nuts from the aisle and pop some into your mouth when you're bored, for at least a palmful a day. Your magnesium, manganese, omega 3 level will improve. And more tomatoes for lycopene and potent prostate friendly meal.

The first prong - Removing inflammation

Cancer is inflammation. You heard that right. Cancer is inflammation. Imagine a wall of fire around your organ. That is as close to how you will get to describing what is going on in your body. While there are many theories of what short-term benefits a little inflammation holds for your body, this is not the good kind of inflammation. This inflammation will mutate your DNA, and cause your cancer to spread and grow beyond its original boundaries into stage 3 and stage 4 forms. The good thing about prostate cancer is that it is slow growing form of cancer, that could take years to get aggressive. And no matter what stage you are in, you can slow it down, degrade it or diminish it all together, that is, if you first remove all sources of inflammation. And herein lies the first prong of the three-pronged approach on the path to wellness. You have to bring down those walls of fire before you cross the moat to the castle that you are about to retake from the enemy !

The first source of inflammation is processed foods. These foods contain food you can eat with a heaping dose of preservatives, nitrites, excito-toxins and stuff you wouldn't need if you actually made your own meal. According to Dr Russell Blaylock, substances that enhance your taste buds, called excito-toxins, called so because they excite your brain cells to death include MSG(monosodium glutamate) a known taste enhancer that is used to the level of 800 lbs a year in US processed foods, and its cousins made the same way in a lab - autolyzed yeast extract, hydrolyzed soy protein, carrageenan. You can make the most disgusting tasting food and dump a load of MSG in it and your taste buds will crave it. MSG is the work horse of the processed food industry. Excito-toxins not only excite your brain cells to death with excess glutamate, while easily crossing the blood-brain barrier, they also add to obesity levels and keep the bad gut bacteria happy by feeding them with more junk food. Needless to say, you want to avoid processed food with MSG or its many named cousins used to "enhance"" taste. That would exclude most processed food except for newer varieties of processed food whose labels actually take pains to show that they do not include these in the ingredients. But alas, those are made using sunflower and other vegetable oils which also increase inflammation by skewing the Omega 6 ratio poorly so it ends up being bad for not just your prostate but also your heart.

The second source is restaurant and fast food. We're talking the use of oil reheated many times over to cook and fry your foods, the use of food colors and binding agents, the materials used to make your food more presentable and all that useless junk that does a lot for aesthetics but precious little for your actual sustenance and health. Reused cooking oil heated and reheated many times is a natural carcinogen so those fried foods you are eating are adding a heaping dose of cancer to your body that your body is already having trouble fighting off. If there is one form of food I would advise you to cut immediately while fighting cancer - this is it - all forms of fried foods. Notice, you don't have to give up on red meat. I like some red meat myself and I like some quickly preparable dishes myself honed through hours of watching those youtube videos. The safest oils to use are olive oils and other fruit oils (coconut, etc) - avoid all vegetable oils as they increase Omega 6s in the body that means more inflammation. Any skew in the Omega 6 to Omega 3 ratio must be made up by more Omega 3 and you really can't eat a tankful of seafood to make up on the increased Omega 6 on a daily basis. So ditch the vegetable oils, please. Stick to the fruit oils.

Eggs are also a source of inflammation for the prostate. If you have a habit of eating at least one egg a day, it might seem a good thing and its probably safe for your health not to exceed that amount. Here's the bad news, even if you consume cage free eggs at one a day - you are increasing your chances of prostate cancer 200% according to new studies. Today's chicken is grown in 6 weeks instead of 9 months with the help of growth hormones. Red meat is actually safer at this point if you stick to using grass fed beef - no hormones, and raised on pasture not corn. The same white meat that sends growth hormones the chicken was injected with into your own body can not only increase your chances of prostate cancer but also increase your partner's chances of breast cancer. Those growth hormones are bad news, much like anabolic steroids. Eat less 'chikin' unless you know the source is organic. Besides, doesn't beef and steak taste better than white meat ? You just want to restrict the red meat to 2-3 meals a WEEK, and substitute more cold water fish so you get your protein intake. At the beginning I would suggest you stop all red meat and focus on getting better first and introduce the meat again in moderate amounts, step by step. In my case I did not have to wait long between stopping meat and restarting it in small amounts - a few months of the three pronged approach was all it took. And during this short time in between treatment and mostly "cured", I had also stopped consuming all eggs which were once my favorite foods to have.

So I am not asking you to cut meat for good. The average American adult is said to consume 100 lbs of meat a year. Yet, meat is not the problem. Not even red meat. The problem is the source and the AMOUNT of red meat you consume. Take it from me, after signs that my prostate cancer was disappearing, I had willy nilly added red meat to a few meals a week, just not to excess. The difference is I knew the source and I moderated well what I ate. I was also in peak shape at the time and today I continue to maintain my muscularity and athleticism at 6” 2”. In the end I sacrificed none of my cravings for a little meat every now and then.

Restricting calories - win-win for all

Restricting calories to 2300-2500 a day will come naturally with these changes. As you offload on sugary snacks, processed foods and consume more home meals and beans and nuts and probiotics, the pangs of hunger in between meals will lessen which will be a win-win both for your waist size and the fight against cancer that you are going to win. Unnecessary calories will only feed cancer cells. Cancer cells just love sugar, especially processed sugar they feed off them and proliferate. With a decent calorie intake not more than what is necessary, you can bring down their food source. And that too without following any new diet fads like ketogenic diets or anything of that sort that are difficult to follow and keep track of, on a daily basis. After all, aren't we here to tell you how to do all this with simple changes Nothing drastic is needed to beat cancer. A slow shift to a healthy lifestyle is all that is needed.

The calorie restricted diet is naturally anti-obesity. While you are beating cancer, you will look better, feel better, feel less lethargic, experience less brain fog and have more energy. Now who wouldn't want that? Trust, me the cavalry you have going in your gut is on your side. They want to see you succeed so they can proliferate. As for the flip side, the bad guys also want to proliferate and would like for you to eat more sugary foods so they can overwhelm the good guys and take over. And you don't want to let that happen. So count your calories by keeping a small book. An example is given below - you can mark the dates you take every food and drink that passes into your mouth for a month or so and then your mind will take over unconsciously and you will not need to keep entries after the first 3 weeks or a month. Experts say that it takes only 21 days or less to build a new habit. And this record keeping is a good habit you can stop in three weeks or continue for the rest of your life. And it only takes few minutes a day. An example of a record is below. In my case you will see I also count proteins with calories as I am also into keeping fit with a minimum protein intake that comes to 140 grams a day for my weight of 200 lbs at my height. While that BMI might be slightly higher than recommended, I am in good health at the time of writing with excellent blood glucose and cholesterol levels in the normal range.

Sample food (lunch, protein in grams)

protein in a glass of milk - 8 gm	Calories - 122
Jarrow's protein scoop - 18 gm x 2 scoops	Calories - 188
protein per tortilla - 3 gm	Calories - 150
Protein per egg - 6 gm	Calories - 66
protein per cup oatmeal - 6 gm	Calories - 300
protein per falafel ball - 2.25 gm	Calories - 57
protein per ounce of beef - 7 gm	Calories - 71
protein per 2 ounces salmon - 11.35 gm	Calories - 118
protein per 0.5 cup of yoghurt - 4.5 gm	Calories - 118
protein per cup of tea(not sweet) - 2 gm	Calories - 30
protein per cup of brown rice - 4.5 gm	Calories - 216
protein per cup of bread - 2 gm	Calories - 70
protein per tbsp sugar - 0 gm	Calories - 48
protein per 1/4 cup sauerkraut - 0 gm	Calories - 5

TOTAL = 94.5 gm	Calories = 1501

Sample food (next day meal, protein in grams)

Egg(1) - 6 gm	Calories - 66
Cup oatmeal(1) - 6 gm	Calories - 300
Milk (1 serving) - 8 gm	Calories - 122
Jarrow's scoop(2) - 36 gm	Calories - 198
Small fish(1 serving) - 10 gm	Calories - 120
Beef(3 oz) - 22 gm	Calories - 223
Tea (2 cups) 3 gm	Calories - 156
Tortillas(3) - 9 gm	Calories - 450
TOTAL = 100 gm	Calories = 1635

Sample food (another day meal, protein in grams)

Egg(1) - 6 gm	Calories - 66
Cup oatmeal(1) - 6 gm	Calories - 300
Milk (1 serving) - 8 gm	Calories - 122
Hummus (45 gm) - 2.2 gm	Calories - 81
Lean scoop(2) - 40 gm	Calories - 300
Beef(6 oz) - 44 gm	Calories - 446
Tea (2 cups) - 3 gm	Calories - 156
Tortillas(2) - 6 gm	Calories - 300
TOTAL = 148.2 gm	Calories = 1690

New studies show that calorie restriction has beneficial effects on the MTOR(mammalian target of rapamycin) signaling pathway. What that means is that an MTOR proteins increase which has been implicated in cancer tumor growth can be slowed down by reducing the calories needed each day. Even a small reduction in calories goes a long way and is life enhancing. The average man over 40 needs only 2300-2500 calories a day while the average woman needs about 1800-2000 calories. By keeping a calorie worksheet like the one above and protein too if you are into fitness, you can keep track of where you are overeating or where you can substitute fruits that actually add negative calories to your diet simply by the energy expended to consume them.

The MTOR or mammalian target of rapamycin was discovered by mistake when studying the immunosuppressant effects of rapamycin on rats. The studies showed that rats showed less signaling along the MTOR pathway and tumors grow more slowly or tumor growth got arrested altogether. Scientists have found that too little MTOR and too much MTOR are both detrimental to human health in that too little MTOR increases ageing while too much MTOR has been implicated in tumor growth.

So with all these benefits for simply bringing down calorie consumption to an acceptable level, would you not agree that the benefits far outweigh the need to eat as one likes even when the body no longer needs such consumption ?

So restricting calories - win-win for all. You'll live longer with or without cancer.

Exercise is important

If you can exercise about 30 minutes a day at least 3 times a week or 45 minutes 2 times a week or 12 minutes every day of the week with many youtube videos available, even better, Exercise slows down cancer. You could get a kettlebell and work out for 10 minutes using it in creative different ways that will leave you stronger and healthier feeling and you will be able to tackle the day better with this small investment of 10 minutes. Besides it will also turn out well for your cancer fighting routine. And you don't need a gym membership to get kicking on kettlebells when there are many youtube videos today showing you just how to do that - chi chi fitness is one good source on youtube.

Get yourself a 10 lb or 12 lb kettlebell or as much as you can handle safely without injury and start today. Even pushups against your own body weight help. Or go to the gym instead for inspiration. Anything and everything in daily movement will work.

Exercise increases the power of your immune system, is a feel good factor in your life and costs little, whether you decide to go to a gym or work out in your own home, using your own body weight or equipment, free or machine. The benefits of exercise extend to fighting cancer as it also improves the MTOR signaling pathway, causes a better regulation of MTOR proteins in the body that has been implicated in tumor growth. So exercise when you can, using some weight to work against for better muscle tone and improved health. Also exercise is a great stress beater and less stress is also considered important as part of your toolkit for fighting cancer. Remember stress is ALSO a source of unwanted inflammation as I explained in chapter 1. Keeping down inflammation is the first barrier in fighting cancer successfully. If you are not keeping down inflammation, you will have to add more resources to the fight against cancer whether that's in the form of more cancer fighting food, medicines or something else. So why not take out the stress when you can with some feel good exercise every now and then. We are talking only about 2-3 days a week, if you can't get time to do anymore than that. Get moving!

Lies, damn lies and statistics

Contrary to popular opinion, FDA approved drugs are not 100% safe. Typically a drug will go through three phases before approval. The sample human population in phase 1 and phase 2 is very, very small typically in tens of patients. At phase 3 the number of patients can be anywhere from a little more higher than in phase 1 and 2 to thousands, but typically in the hundreds assuming such patients can be found and willing to be experimented on with the new drug. Any new drug being developed has its efficacy and safety compared to patients taking the standard regimen of an earlier approved drug in the same category.

Take the example of figitumumab, an experimental drug developed by Pfizer used to treat a particular form of lung cancer. It was eventually rejected because its safety fell below that of the standard regimen drug at 5% vs 1% treatment-related deaths. This means the standard regimen still had a treatment related death rate of 1 in 100 lung cancer patients! No doubt, that one patient would most likely have been someone like me, given my adverse reaction to most drugs. Now you see why I'm not too elated about being a statistic related drug death. There are lies, damn lies and then there are statistics. No doubt if the other 99 patients did not die, they would suffer side effects that would be considered passable for the treatment benefit. That said, no drug would be approved by the FDA if they required a 100% safety record and the costs of developing a drug till they had a 100% safety record in phase 3 would be astronomical, to put it lightly. So the statistic of 99 in 100 not being killed by the drug treatment in the standard regimen case was considered passable for use as a standard against newer drugs being developed.

Just not passable for me.

Ten micronutrients to beat cancer

The ten important nutrients are l-lysine, vitamin C, proline, copper, manganese, NAC, selenium, quercetin, EGCG (there's that green tea again), and l-arginine.

A doctor, scientist, and humanitarian named Matthias Rath placed a full-page ad in USA Today with the provocative headline, "Breakthrough in Cancer Research." In it, the German-born scientist explained that a safe, effective, all-natural, scientifically-proven approach to controlling the spread of cancer has been found.

This pioneering and outspoken scientist continues to seek out safe and effective natural treatments, particularly for the most deadly forms of cancer, and he doesn't mince words as far as drug companies are concerned: "These economic powers are determined to sacrifice the lives of millions of people for profits."

Matthias Rath researched heart disease in the 1980s and found a link with vitamin C. After reading his findings in the

American Heart Association journal Arteriosclerosis in 1987, double Nobel prize-winning scientist Linus Pauling -- best known for popularizing vitamin C -- invited Dr. Rath to join him in the US, which he did three years later.

When Dr. Pauling died in 1994, he went on to form the Dr. Rath Research Institute in California, a 23,000 square foot pharmaceutical grade laboratory with particular emphasis on the benefits of micronutrients in cancer. Dr. Rath and his long-standing associate Dr. Aleksandra Niedzwiecki believe cancer is no longer a mysterious illness. The key mechanisms by which it develops and can be controlled are now easily understood.

Since nine out of ten patients die because cancer has spread from the primary organ to other parts of the body, they focused their attention on these metastases, as they're called. Cancer develops into a life-threatening illness because the tumor is able to escape its confinement. It does so by mimicking a process that happens naturally in a healthy body.

Why tumors grow more frequently in certain organs

Cells are kept in position because they are surrounded by connective tissue made up of various fibers such as collagen and elastin. But sometimes this needs to be loosened to allow cells, fluids or other material to move through. For instance, during the menstrual cycle a mature egg must pass through the ovary wall and make its journey to the womb. To achieve this, hormones signal the production of collagen-digesting enzymes to momentarily dissolve the connective tissue.

The body also needs to produce these enzymes to allow immune cells to reach their target and when any kind of tissue remodeling is required, such as when breast tissue is prepared for lactation. Other processes that use these collagen-digesting enzymes include wound healing and body growth. For example, they are highly active in bone growth in the young.

Like an automatic door that opens just as you approach it and then closes behind when you've passed through, in a healthy body this is a precisely timed and tightly regulated process. But cancer cells hijack this mechanism, using it for their own purposes to digest tissue continually in an uncontrolled manner. The immune system sees this as a normal process and does nothing to stop it, while the body's own enzyme inhibitors are insufficient to stop cancer's onward march.

Drs. Rath and Niedzwiecki believe this process answers the question as to why cancer forms in some organs and systems more frequently than others. It's because the more vulnerable organs already use collagen-digesting enzymes under normal circumstances. These are the breast, ovary, uterus, cervix, testes, prostate, bones (especially in children and adolescents), and white blood cells (involved in leukemia).

These are more susceptible to connective tissue digestion getting out of control and so are more prone to cancer. The same collagen-digesting mechanism applies during metastasis. Cancer cells are able to "puncture" the network of small blood vessels (capillaries) that surround them and enter the bloodstream. The more a cancer cell is able to produce these enzymes, the more aggressive the cancer will be, the faster it will spread, and the shorter the life expectancy of the patient -- unless the process can be stopped.

Natural ways to block collagen-digesting enzymes

Although the body's internal systems are unable to stop ongoing connective tissue destruction by cancer cells, nature itself provides us with substances to slow down or stop it. The most important is the essential amino acid L-lysine. Our daily requirement is greater than any other amino acid. It comprises 12% of the elastin and collagen mass. A person weighing 155 pounds would have 1.3 pounds of lysine in their body.

Not only is it an essential building block of collagen, but lysine will also – if there's enough of it -- occupy sites where collagen-digesting enzymes bind to connective tissue molecules to inhibit tissue degradation.

Vitamin C – which we also need to get from our food -- stimulates collagen and elastin production and contributes to strong connective tissue.

Proline, an amino acid the body is able to make in limited amounts, is another important building block of collagen.

Copper and manganese are also essential for collagen formation, while N-acetyl cysteine (NAC), the green tea extract Epigallocatechin Gallate (EGCG) and quercetin, act synergistically to strengthen the connective tissue. The mineral selenium is able to inhibit connective tissue digestion.

Most of these nutrients also have many other anti-cancer effects.

Scientific proof

Dr. Rath and his colleagues carried out a test on human prostate cells in culture to find out whether their micronutrient formula could block the secretion of two collagen-digesting enzymes used by cancer cells. In both cases, the higher the concentration of micronutrients, the lower the production of these enzymes. In the case of both enzymes, moderate and higher levels of micronutrients stopped their secretion completely. This was later confirmed in 40 types of human cancer.

The next test was to see if micronutrients could stop cancer cells from penetrating connective tissue. Here the scientists used a vial with a membrane of connective tissue in the middle. Below it was a solution that mimicked human body fluid. Above it was the same fluid containing human cancer cells. Other vials were prepared, identical to the first, except that different levels of micronutrients were added to the upper chambers with the tumor cells.

While all cancer cells successfully penetrated the connective tissue in the first vial, as micronutrient concentrations increased, so did their ability to prevent cancer invasion until -- at the highest concentration – cancer cells were totally blocked, with none found in the lower half of the vial.

For some types of tumor this total blockade was achieved at low micronutrient concentrations. For others it took moderate or high levels to achieve the same result. Altogether, Dr. Rath and his colleagues demonstrated this effect in all of the 40 different types of human cancer tested.

In their ebook Victory Over Cancer, Drs. Rath and Niedzwiecki write, "Some chemotherapy proponents may argue that the solution to cancer cannot be that simple. But it can – and we know why: All cancer cells use the same mechanism to invade the surrounding tissue and metastasize. Since micronutrients are capable of blocking this universal cellular mechanism, they can inhibit the invasion of any type of cancer cells irrespective of their origin."

It works in animal studies

After injecting a group of mice with melanoma cells, they were divided into three groups. The first were given a normal diet only (control). The second had micronutrients added to the diet. The mice in the third group were given micronutrients by injection into the bloodstream.

When the researchers measured metastasis to the lungs, they found it was reduced by 60% in the second group compared to the controls. This increased to 80% in the intravenous group. To take this research even further, the scientists carried out a study that more accurately reflects how cancer progresses in humans.

This time they injected melanoma cells into the spleens of two groups of mice, one eating a normal diet and the other the same thing with micronutrients added. The result was significantly less tumor growth in the supplemented group. When the researchers checked the liver -- the main target for the spread of melanoma -- they found metastases reduced by almost half compared to the controls. Melanoma is generally a very aggressive form of cancer.

Micronutrients block four mechanisms

While metastasis is the Rath team's main focus, cancer cells also grow by multiplying, forming new blood vessels (angiogenesis) and by not responding to normal cell signals to self-destruct (apoptosis). So they repeated the previous tests and found supplemented mice had significantly smaller tumors. The scientists wrote that "the results were amazing." Growth was inhibited in ten human tumors tested, with reductions ranging from 36% in liver cancer to 78% in breast cancer over a period of just four weeks.

Tumors as little as 1/25th of an inch cannot grow without forming new blood vessels to provide their own blood supply. This process is dependent on the use of collagen-digesting enzymes. For this reason the scientists were confident that angiogenesis could be inhibited.

They were right. Exposing cultured human endothelial cells to increasing amounts of micronutrients, they found the more that were added, the less capillary structures were formed. At the highest micronutrient concentration the process was completely blocked.

According to the authors, "This study is irrefutable scientific proof that micronutrients are powerful anti-angiogenic agents that can be immediately applied to help control cancer." Next they tested whether micronutrients can induce apoptosis. L-arginine was included in the micronutrient mix because it is a precursor to nitric oxide. A deficiency of arginine can limit the production of this molecule, which has been shown to act as an inducer of apoptosis.

Here again they met with success. The higher the concentration of micronutrients added to melanoma cells, the more they underwent natural death. At the highest concentration, virtually all cells died naturally. This means -- if it applies not only in the lab but in the human body -- that micronutrients can reverse existing tumors.

According to Dr. Rath, this mix of natural compounds

works at a genetic level to convert cancer cells that are immortal to ones that start dying. Micronutrients go to the core of the cancer cell -- to its DNA-- essentially "giving orders" to function properly or die.

Results in cancer patients

In Europe, where Dr. Rath now lives and is much better known, more than 10,000 patients have used or are using his synergistic micronutrient program. If cancer has progressed too far or if patients have been subject to intensive chemotherapy -- which cripples the immune system -- then recovery may not be possible.

However, many patients have now survived 15 years beyond their predicted death. Dr Rath has medical documentation on many of them. One of these is Werner Pilniok, who was diagnosed with a fast growing lung tumor in 1999 at the age of 68 and given six months to live. After reading about Dr. Rath's research, he canceled surgery and opted for large quantities of the recommended micronutrients instead. Six months later he had a CT scan. The cancer was gone. His oncologist was astonished. She could not believe her eyes. Mr Pilniok celebrated his 80th birthday in 2011 and was still known to be alive in 2015.

Another remarkable case was Ilona Schmidt, who was diagnosed with a brain tumor. Her conventional doctors administered radiation treatment and prescribed cortisone. She said, "I wanted to die at that time, I felt so terrible." The treatments did not help and the doctors gave her no hope of survival. She started following Dr. Rath's protocol in April 2002. Shortly after this she was taken off cortisone. In September of the same year, an MRI scan confirmed that the tumor had vanished. In an interview, Dr. Rath said, "There is no program that we are aware of in the field of natural health that is more effective in controlling cancer."

To sum up, the ten food based cancer fighting nutrients

are l-lysine, vitamin C, proline, copper, manganese, NAC, selenium, quercetin, EGCG, and l-arginine. Personally I take some of these like Vitamin C(daily 500 mg), NAC(every now and then), quercetin(daily 500 mg), EGCG(as green tea every now and then). Pick and choose what you think will be beneficial to you - you don't have to take everything with my three pronged approach doing most of the work.

Moringa olefeira killer superfood

There's one plant that really does live up to the superfood label. It's packed with good nutrition and contains compounds with powerful healing and anti-cancer properties. It's called moringa. And it can help protect you against hundreds of diseases. Also known as horseradish tree, drumstick tree, benzolive tree and ben oil tree, moringa is native to the Himalayan foothills (northern India, Pakistan and Nepal) and widely cultivated in tropical and subtropical countries.

Moringa is a genus with 13 different species, but the best known is Moringa oleifera. This is the variety most commonly used as food and medicine, and also the one most studied. Its use can be traced back 4000 years, and according to India's traditional Ayurvedic medicine, moringa can prevent 300 diseases.

Traditional use includes improving alertness, maintaining healthy skin, healing skin infections, enhancing energy, relieving pain, aiding digestion, combating anxiety and stress, and treating wounds, warts, asthma, dental decay, fever, diarrhea, gout, high blood pressure, diabetes, inflammation, tumors and sore throats.

Traditional medicine uses all parts of the plant, for different purposes, but it's the leaves that are used most often in nutritional supplements. When you pop a moringa supplement, you get a dose of all essential amino acids – the ones we have to get from our food because our bodies don't make them.

Moringa also boasts an abundance of vitamins, with especially high concentrations of vitamins A and C, and a wide range of minerals, trace elements and assorted plant chemicals most of us never heard of – but which are probably the most important reason for consuming moringa, because we can get the minerals, amino acids and vitamins elsewhere. For these reasons, some authorities call moringa the most nutrient-rich of all plants.

Potent antioxidant and broad-spectrum healer

Moringa also contains a large number of compounds with strong antioxidant activity. Writing in the Journal of Medicinal Food in 2010, researchers stated: "The high antioxidant/radical scavenging effects observed for different parts of M. oleifera appear to provide justification for their widespread therapeutic use in traditional medicine in different continents. The possibility that this high antioxidant/radical scavenging capacity may impact on the cancer chemopreventive potential of the plant must be considered."

As well as being a powerful antioxidant, other mechanisms of action are described by Memorial Sloan Kettering Cancer Center. Normally not a friend of alternatives, this mainstream medical institute lists the following benefits derived from laboratory studies. The plant:

- lowers high blood fats and cholesterol
- counters atherosclerosis and helps prevent heart disease
- protects the liver and kidneys
- reduces elevated blood sugar and improves glucose tolerance
- is anti-inflammatory via several different mechanisms
- is antibacterial, antiviral, antifungal and antiparasitic
- blocks pain
- suppresses an overactive immune response
- has antisickling activity (lowers the risk of sickle cell anemia, an inherited disease among some people of African descent)
- prevents bladder and urinary tract stone formation
- offers protection from stomach ulcers and alleviates symptoms of ulcerative colitis
- balances hormones
- shows protective effects against Alzheimer's disease
- promotes wound healing
- acts against cancer

With this vast array of health benefits, it's easy to see why moringa is dubbed the "miracle tree". Moringa contains a rare, unique and diverse combination of plant compounds. About 110 have been identified from the whole genus. Of these, 88 are from the oleifera species alone. It’s truly impressive.

An anticancer cocktail

Many of these compounds possess anti-cancer activity. The following are just a handful of examples found in the leaves.

Quercetin: Researchers at Boston University School of Medicine found this flavonoid inhibited the growth of some types of malignant cells "and also displays unique anticancer properties."

Kaempferol: A comprehensive review published in Phytotherapy Research in November described this flavonoid as having "a significant role in reducing cancer" through a range of mechanisms including apoptosis (inducing cell suicide), and down=regulating various signaling and protein expression pathways. Kaempferol is by no means common, so moringa is a good place to get a dose.

Genistein: Wayne State University scientists describe this isoflavone, normally found in soy products, as a potent inhibitor of angiogenesis (blood vessels formed by cancer cells to promote their growth) and metastasis, with "multi-targeted biological and molecular effects in cancer cells." If you prefer to avoid soy, moringa is a good place to get genistein.

Myricetin: This flavonoid was described by Chinese scientists writing in Oncology Letters as being "significantly effective in the treatment of various types of cancers, including prostate cancer, hepatocellular [liver] carcinoma, gastric cancer and human squamous cell carcinoma." I never heard of it prior to preparing this article, so moringa is your ticket.

Ellagic acid: Scientists from the University of Rome have just published a review of this polyphenolic compound in "Nutrients". They describe its anticancer effects in culture and rodent models against colorectal, breast, prostate, lung, melanoma, bladder, liver, ovarian, oral, brain and bone cancer. It works through multiple mechanisms to stop the growth and spread of tumors. We've noted before that ellagic acid is available in raspberries, but eating them every day is probably beyond most of us. Consider moringa.

Moringa cancer studies

Between 2008 and 2017, ten studies have looked at the anti-cancer effects of Moringa oleifera extracts mainly derived from the leaf, but also the bark and seeds, on human cancer cell lines. This is not as good as tests on live animals or humans, but it's indicative, and many of us take certain supplements on the basis of such in vitro or test tube studies. Moringa was effective at inhibiting the growth of cancers of the lung, liver, pancreas, breast, colorectum, prostate and blood.2

Of the many active compounds found in Moringa oleifera, some of the most important are the isothiocyanates. They're being actively researched for their many biological activities including anti-inflammatory, antidiabetic and antimicrobial effects as well as anticancer.

Described as a "potent anticancer compound," isothiocyanates extracted from oleifera leaf extract were shown to induce apoptosis in a number of different cancer cells. This could "open new frontiers in cancer therapeutics." As well as isothiocyanates, Moringa oleifera was found to inhibit cancer cell proliferation mainly due to a phenolic compound called eugenol, and a rare naturally-occurring sugar called D-allose.

Eugenol targets E2F1, a protein that is overexpressed in many cancers, and another protein, survivin, that stimulates cancer growth. D-allose was found to have "a significant inhibitory effect on cancer cell proliferation." Chemotherapy works better with moringa

Most patients are on the lookout for natural remedies they can do at the same time as chemotherapy. Be aware that many oncologists will still oppose the use of ANY supplements. A research group from India investigated whether Moringa oleifera leaf extract could offer protection against the toxic effects of chemotherapy. Administered prior to the drug in mice, they reported improvements in male gonad function after the procedure. They concluded that the extract "may have potential benefit in reducing the loss of male gonadal function following chemotherapy."

Another study looked at whether the plant could offer protection from bladder damage, which is known to be caused by the chemotherapy drug cyclophosphamide (CP). The researchers found that "Moringa leaves play an important role in ameliorating and protecting the bladder from CP toxicity." When Moringa oleifera leaf extract was combined with the chemotherapy drug doxorubicin and tested on an immortal human cell line used in research called HeLa, the combination produced a better outcome than the drug alone. Reviewing all these findings, a research group wrote, "The application of currently used anticancer drugs combined with M. oleifera could be a novel therapeutic strategy for cancers."

How to take Moringa

Moringa can be found in many forms. The oil from the

seeds in used in skin creams, lotions and soap. Whole seeds can be purchased, and dried leaves are used to produce moringa tea. There are even some energy bars that incorporate the leaf powder. Moringa powder has been described as having a pleasant, earthy, spinachy flavor. It can be sprinkled on salads, soups or blended into a smoothie. Not everyone is enamored with the taste, however, so some people prefer to take it in capsules. The usual dose is 500 to 1000 milligrams a day.

Dangers of antibiotics .... in animals

There is a tricky but essential thing to avoid in the meat you buy. Organic food is better for you than non-organic, because it's always better to keep pesticides and herbicides out of your body.

Another reason to eat organic is to avoid the antibiotics that are frequently found in meat. These drugs are fed to animals because apparently they promote quick weight gain, and also enable cattle and chickens to survive the extremely unhealthy conditions on factory farms. The animals are overcrowded and the pens are filthy.

The animals that receive antibiotics are dosed regularly – sometimes even daily. The drugs are mixed in with their food and water, a practice known as sub-therapeutic administration. When you eat these animals, you're taking the drugs just as surely as if you popped a pill from a prescription bottle. Antibiotics may be life-saving substances if you actually have a bacterial infection that your immune system can't handle on its own. But when they're in your grilled steak, scrambled eggs or baked chicken they don't benefit you in any way.

You want to avoid these unwanted drugs, but to do that you need to know a few tricks of the agriculture trade. Otherwise you'll end up eating drug-tainted food you thought was pure. If you know about this issue, you already know that feeding antibiotics to farm animals has given rise to superbugs. These are selected bacteria that survive the antibiotics while the weak strains of bacteria die. The survivors breed and thrive, resulting in antibiotic-resistant bacteria that few or no drugs can kill.

These superbugs are showing up in our meat sources and lead to food poisoning outbreaks caused by MRSA in pork and resistant salmonella in turkey, to name just a couple of examples. But you probably don't know there's an even more sinister effect of antibiotic abuse: the increased risk of cancer and other life-threatening diseases.

Meat and poultry producers in the U.S. aren't required to report how they use drugs on their livestock. Meaning we don't know how much and which animals are getting the heaviest doses... yet hundreds of millions of us eat the meat that comes out of those farms.

Because of the non-reporting -- and for various other reasons -- it's hard to directly connect the spread of superbugs to overuse of antibiotics in livestock. Regardless, the Centers for Disease Control and Prevention (CDC) and other government agencies have testified before Congress that there's a clear link, and powerful groups like the American Academy of Pediatrics, and the American Medical Association all agree.

But for the moment, let's leave aside the issue of antibiotic-resistant bacteria. How might eating antibiotics every day in meat directly affect us? Very likely it affects our gut microbiomes. The constant carpet bombing by antibiotics must kill the friendly bacteria in our digestive tract.

The collection of bacteria in your gut microbiome is one of

the leading indicators of immune system health. With a wide-ranging, thriving, diverse garden of gut bacteria, your immune system functions at its best, inflammation levels stay down, and the threat of killer diseases like cancer stays at bay. But without a diverse microbiome, your immune system isn't as efficient. You're more likely to face inflammation. And overall, you're more likely to develop cancer and other diseases.

Clarity and standards remain murky

So what's an omnivore to do? If you want to keep meat in your diet but avoid antibiotics, you can begin with reading labels – though even those are baffling. For example, buying fish can be confusing. As yet there are no USDA organic standards for farmed fish. That means fish may be labeled "organic" despite treatment with antibiotics. There are no rules. Fish farmers regularly use antibiotics, and over a third of the world's seafood is farmed.

As far as eggs go, regulations permit fewer antibiotics for egg-laying chickens. That's reassuring, but studies have found antibiotic residues in eggs despite reports from the poultry industry that antibiotic use is limited. And a 2000 study from the Journal of Agricultural and Food Chemistry showed antibiotics can linger for some time in a chicken's eggs.

And then here are some labels that don't tell you anything useful: Natural, Antibiotic-Free, and No Antibiotic Residues. The first only means nothing has been added to the meat itself, after the slaughter (like artificial color). Antibiotics could still have been used while the animal was alive. In fact, "Natural" is an unregulated term that may mean nothing at all. And the terms "Antibiotic-Free" and "No Antibiotic Residues" aren't authorized or regulated by the USDA. So they too can mean anything and everything - or nothing.

Labels to look for and look past

The standards are stricter for meat. If a food producer

wants to use the organic seal from the Department of Agriculture, it has to agree not to give antibiotics to animals raised for meat. But there are exceptions. For example, chickens and turkeys can receive antibiotics on their first day of life and still be considered "organic."

So if you want to be sure your poultry is completely free of antibiotics, you'll want to look for a "raised without antibiotics" label along with the "organic" label. Another reassuring label to look for is the "USDA Process Verified" seal on the meat package. It means USDA inspectors visited the farm and confirmed that no antibiotics were used.

Eat out less. Screen the meat you buy and cook. Easy peasy.

Optimizing your diet based on methylation

Diet plans are a big industry, and it seems hundreds of people stump for different kinds of diets. In the world of alternative health, the most popular options these days are the keto, Paleo and vegetarian eating plans.

And while a lot of people are still searching for that holy grail of a diet that will fix all their problems, my reading and personal experience suggest that no single diet is best for everyone. Each of us is unique when it comes to body chemistry.

So it's good news to know one field of scientific study – based on your genes -- has started to capitalize on individual diet needs – to the point where it may help you figure out which diet really is best for you to eat so you look great, feel great, and most importantly, keep illnesses like cancer at bay.

Can your DNA determine what you eat?

"Nutrigenetics" is the name of this new science. Its goal is to figure out which gene variants are associated with different responses to different nutrients, and from there, to relate any variations to diseases like cancer.

We know cancer is a leading killer, and we know different genetic factors play a role in predisposing some individuals to certain cancers. Some of those factors, like gene alterations and DNA instability, are affected by your nutritional intake. A lot of that is because nutrition possibly leads to DNA methylation, or the repression of gene transcription (which has to do with how cells sustain themselves). When this process gets interrupted, possibly because of a lack of nutrition or due to too much of one food or another, then cancer is more likely to occur.

Or, to put it simply, you're predisposed to certain cancers because of your genetics. Whether or not you end up developing those cancers has a lot to do with the nutrition your body receives over time. But we're not all predisposed to the same cancers. The important thing to understand is that if you ARE genetically predisposed to, say, breast cancer or prostate cancer, you can "activate" them or keep them at bay based on nutrition. According to nutrigenetics, the reason is that the type of nutrition we each need varies from one person to another, even when it comes to activating or disabling the same cancer.

Investigating your nutrition-related genes and at-home DNA tests

So – the theory is that nutrigenetics is able to highlight the relationship between nutrition and gene expression. Where do we go from there? For starters – if it's true -- it should help researchers better understand the mechanisms behind cancer, as well as how it develops in the body. Since we have plenty of evidence that shows genetic factors play a role in the development of cancer, and we also know things like DNA instability and gene alterations are affected by what we eat, it makes sense that understanding nutrition-affected genes could be an exciting new frontier.

Yet nutrigenetics is controversial and still has little research behind it. Some researchers argue that most of the genetic variations considered in nutrigenetics are such minor influences that it's potentially not worth looking at. Genes may account for something like ten percent of your cancer risk. They aren't the whole story or even a big part of it.

Now, if nutrigenetics wants to focus on how food affects gene expression, that's a whole different story – and I think it's an exciting one. Epigenetics or gene expression is the science of how external factors – including food – can turn certain genes on or off.

Of course, the companies who are gearing up to sell nutrigenetics test kits would disagree with their critics. DNAFit, a London-based company founded in 2013 that looks at genetic information for fitness and nutrition, is one of them. At present, they sell mouth-swab kits that the customer or practitioner sends to the company's lab in Norwich, England. DNAFit analyses the sample and generates a report on how a person might tailor his or her diet and exercise habits to achieve "optimal fitness. If you can do this type of DNA based tailoring of diet it may be beneficial. Just a thought, another quiver in the arsenal available to you. If this is too expensive and beyond reach, read on. (Spoiler: I did not do this either but I like the possibility of mix- and match approaches like adding to my own three-pronged approaches in the future and you can do the same, tailoring for your needs as you see fit. These are complementary tools, not necessary.)

Undermethylation and cancer risk

It's a big word that you probably don't think applies to you. And your doctor may not even know about it yet. Yet it's becoming the latest buzzword in natural health – and for good reason. Methylation affects your ability to think, repair DNA, turn genes on and off, fight infections, and get rid of environmental toxins, just for starters. Without it, you wouldn't be alive.

Methylation occurs in your body more than a billion times per second. Suffice it to say, anything that happens a billion times per second is probably worth knowing about, since it's clearly "mission critical." In this case, we're talking about a vital biochemical process that occurs when one molecule passes a methyl group (one carbon atom plus 3 hydrogen atoms, CH_3) to another molecule.

Through this process, your body makes cysteine, taurine, sulfate, creatine, carnitine, CoQ10, phosphatidylcholine, melatonin, and tons of other important substances. Methylation also causes your body to produce ATP, your cells' primary energy unit. ATP is the end-product of mitochondria, the cell's "batteries" or "energy factories." Take ATP out of the picture, and nothing works well.

But two major factors affect how well your body methylates – genetics and environment.

Half of us have defective methylation and most of us probably don't even know there's a problem. Nor do our doctors, in most cases. Scientific literature refers to methylation SNP's (pronounced "snips") as genetic "defects" – though it might be more accurate to call them a "genetic personality." SNP's breed methyl-folate deficiencies, which lead to glutathione deficiency and, eventually, to toxic buildup in your blood and tissues.

Glutathione's nickname is "master antioxidant." It's critical to detoxification, among other things. A deficiency can leave you wide open to infection, and result in chronic fatigue, fibromyalgia, autoimmune disease, multiple chemical sensitivities, and many progressive diseases.

This SNP in particular has created a lot of buzz

An estimated 45 to 55 percent of people have the genetic mutation MTHFR (revealed by testing). Methylation is part of a complex metabolic cycle involving coordinated action by multiple enzymes. Mutations such as the MTHFR mean decreased enzyme activity – and, by default, decreased methylation.

You can inherit the MTHFR defect from both parents or from just one. Having two copies of a mutated gene is considerably higher risk and can be fatal, compared to having one non-mutated copy of the gene and one mutated copy.

You can find out if you have this defect at www.23andMe.com, the company that directly provides consumers information about their genome without a doctor's prescription. I have done this test and found that I am homozygous for the MTHFR defect, that is I have this "snip" from both parents. I also have the VDRTaq SNP, which makes more likely the possibility of defective processing of Vitamin D so I supplement my Vit D at 5000 IU per day which has supported me in the fight against cancer as well as contributed greatly to my overall immunity to COVID and other respiratory illnesses.

You might've heard that the FDA came down on this company several years ago for failing to comply with various regulations concerning "medical devices." But you can still get the raw data by taking their saliva test, then going to www.GeneticGenie.org for your report. Your functional doctor can help you interpret it.

Knowing this information can save your life

Methylation affects your entire body – including your immune system, brain, heart, lungs, skin, GI tract, and endocrine glands. So the ramifications of reduced methylation are significant. If you're positive for MTHFR defect, you'll be prone to folate deficiency, low glutathione, toxic overload and impaired detox capacity, and homocysteine buildup, potentially leading to heart attack or stroke.

Due to immune dysregulation and histamine intolerance, you'll be more susceptible to infections, cancer, and allergies. Methylation defects are also linked to depression, anxiety, chronic fatigue, infertility, miscarriage, and an array of other health issues. But please, don't fall into the trap of thinking one-dimensionally about isolated diseases, as if your body is a disjointed conglomeration of separate organs and functions.

Methylation – hidden key to gene expression?

While you may have never heard of methylation and your doctor may not know much more than you do, understanding its role is critical to gaining and keeping good health. One of methylation's most critical functions is regulating gene expression. It turns your genes on and off (activating and silencing them). A methyl group binds to a gene to change how it expresses... known as DNA methylation.

A couple of decades ago, scientists believed you were stuck with the genes you inherited from your parents. Now we know better. You can do plenty to determine how your genes express themselves. Instead of bemoaning the bad hand you were dealt, it's time to rejoice that you can revise your own health destiny.

It matters to your brain

Methylation plays a key role in making neurotransmitters like sleep-producing melatonin and energy-producing epinephrine. It's important to understand that it's not just the making of neurotransmitters that's important. If you can't also break them down, you could end up with seizure disorders, insomnia, panic attacks, or rage. Scientists believe poor methylation may be linked to autism, ADHD, depression, and even neurodegenerative diseases like Parkinson's and Alzheimer's.

Watch out for these methylation thieves

Any number of issues can disrupt methylation. Some researchers believe nearly everyone suffers from defective methylation. Here are some of the biggest methylation busters:

1. Nutrient deficiencies that reduce the active form of folate in your body – zinc, B2/riboflavin, magnesium, B6, and B12 in the form of methyl-cobalamin, and folate, for example.
2. Poor diet, poor probiotic status, foods (even organic) grown in poor soil, digestive problems, bowel conditions.
3. Environmental chemicals – increase toxicity and increase the body's need for methyl groups.
4. Medications that steal methylation nutrients – methotrexate, metformin, antacids, acid blockers, proton pump inhibitors (Prilosec, Nexium and others), corticosteroids, birth

control pills, and nitrous oxide.

5. Alcohol – slows methylation and depletes the body's supply of glutathione.

6. Green coffee bean extract is high in catechols, which burn through methylation nutrients incredibly fast.

7. Low magnesium reduces methylation. Many people are deficient without knowing it.

8. Heavy metals – mercury in your food or teeth, lead in your bloodstream, cadmium if you smoke, copper or arsenic...

9. High levels of acetyl aldehyde, a potent neurotoxin released by Candida yeast and alcohol.

10. Lyme disease, which you may have without realizing it. The Borrelia burgdorferi germ steals magnesium to make biofilms and hide. This may explain why some "Lymies" have horrific reactions during antibiotic treatment. After the antibiotics, the body is forced to remove the "dead bug parts" and ammonia, which spikes when the drug kills off the Borrelia microbes.

11. Advancing age.

How to improve methylation naturally

Improving methylation could be one of the best things you can do to support your health. And it may be simpler than you think – whether or not you have the MTHFR defect. Don't let your doctor tell you there's nothing you can do to improve your methylation... or that, because it's "genetic," you're stuck with what you have. There are always things you can do.

Your actions could improve your health or even save your life – since this process is linked to so many critical functions and deadly diseases. If your doctor won't work with you, find one who understands methylation and will help you with a protocol.

Worth considering: Some experts believe that certain people over-methylate. Others believe most people have inadequate methylation even with healthy diets, possibly due to poor soil and heavy pollution. It's still controversial. So what can you do? Eat natural foods. Methyl groups are found in quinoa, spinach, lamb, chicken, and beets. Eat lots of lightly cooked dark green leafy veggies. Avoid processed foods and vegan diets.

Methylation enhancing protocol

One of the most effective and least expensive nutrients to enhance production of methyl groups is TMG (trimethylglycine). TMG converts homocysteine into methionine and, in the process, produces natural SAMe, another beneficial nutrient.

TMG is inexpensive, readily available, and also goes by the name glycine betaine. It comes from sugar beets. Note that betaine HCL is another creature altogether. Don't confuse the two. TMG facilitates increased methylation, and not only protects you from disease, but also helps you feel younger.

Studies show that supplementing with folate – NOT folic acid – can help override a methylation defect. Methylation guru Dr. Ben Lynch never recommends folic acid. It's synthetic and may be harmful. Some studies associate it with increased cancer risk.

What else? These all boost glutathione and help methylation:

• Sulfur-containing foods like onion, garlic, kale, broccoli, cauliflower, cabbage, and bok choy.

• Un-denatured whey protein powder (if you tolerate dairy).

• Selenium, 200 mcg per day.

• Exercise. Get out and move your body.

• Sleep. Get 7 to 9 hours per night. Sleep deprivation depletes glutathione.

• Milk thistle, 100 to 300 mg per day. Silymarin is the most recommended form.

• Probiotics – help control Candida and lower toxic acetyl aldehyde.

• Methylated forms of vitamins B6, B9 and B12.

If you learn you have the MTHFR defect, it can feel like

you've been hit with a ton of bricks. The VDRTaq defect is obviously easier to overcome if you have genetically low Vitamin D levels. Arming yourself with this knowledge gives you a chance to rewrite your own health story. That's something your parents and grandparents couldn't even dream of. So take advantage of this knowledge. It makes the fight against cancer that much easier.

Dangers of arachidonic acid

The tricky thing about good health is how much of it relies on the domino effect. For example, say you take a walk in the morning to the coffee shop around the corner. The sunshine and fresh air make you feel good, so you order a smoothie for breakfast, which gives you an energy boost so you're ready for work, which leaves you feeling positive and capable, which translates to swinging by the gym on your way home, followed by a heart-healthy meal and a good nights' sleep.

Sounds like a great day, right? Do this kind of thing regularly, and your overall health either improves or stays good. But let's say it's raining, so you skip your morning walk. You stay home and make yourself bacon and eggs for breakfast. The heavier meal makes you sleepy throughout the day so you're not very productive, which puts you in a bad mood. You grab a burger on your way home, which you eat in front of the TV, followed by on-and-off dozing till you rouse yourself after midnight and finally shuffle to bed.

Do that kind of thing regularly, and your overall health plummets. So it's worth considering the little things that affect your health, and especially the foods that make you happy and energetic versus the foods that bring you down – emotionally and physically. Here's one of the foods that's a bringdown.

You might never suspect it, but eggs can ruin your mood. This is tricky territory, because eggs have come in for pretty good press lately (including by me) – after decades of being trashed by doctors. Whatever their faults, they do contain the "perfect protein." They're easy to cook, readily available, cheap, and high in nutrients... what's not to love?

The answer is something you've probably never heard of: arachidonic acid. It's an inflammatory omega-6 fatty acid your own body produces. So clearly, you need it. In small quantities it's benign, but there's such a thing as too much arachidonic acid. And when you get it in excess, you're at risk for inflammatory diseases and mood disorders.

Besides carrying it in your own body, you'll find arachidonic acid in animal products -- and eggs and poultry in particular. According to Japanese researchers, eating just one egg a day is enough to significantly raise the arachidonic acid levels found in your bloodstream.

Proof you can have too much of a good thing

Early evidence shows arachidonic acid can trigger blain inflammation. This puts you at higher risk of suicide and depression. If you suffer from depression or your family is predisposed to it, this is something to take seriously. On the flipside, epidemiological studies show that eating a diet high in carbohydrates and low in both fat and protein (meaning you consume very little arachidonic acid) correlates with lower levels of anxiety and depression.

We all know about the benefits of a whole food, plant-based diet. In a study that followed overweight or diabetic employees who tried it, the participants had more energy, higher-quality sleep, and improved mental health, at least when compared to a control group of people who ate whatever they wanted.

This study was followed by a similar study at ten different sites where the researchers found comparable improvements in anxiety, depression, and emotional health thanks to a meat-free, plant-based diet. Meat intake should be moderate. For whatever it's worth, my personal approach is to eat meat at maybe two-maximum of three meals a week – and no processed meats such as hot dogs or bacon.

Meat and eggs can accelerate prostate cancer

Here's another fact that can't be denied: arachidonic acid also appears to stimulate the growth of prostate cancer cells by as much as 200 percent. And PSA levels – which are a measure of prostate inflammation – tend to increase exponentially.

Because prostate cancer often grows at a slow rate, older men don't have to worry about it much. They just need to monitor their condition to make sure it doesn't go downhill (about one prostate cancer out of ten is fast-growing). Most men will die of old age before they die of prostate cancer, and the condition is way over-treated in our society.

But if you indulge in a diet heavy in arachidonic acid, the prostate's secretions of PSA will likely skyrocket – and prostate cancer cell growth may accelerate. I would venture that if you KNOW you have a prostate tumor and you've adopted the "watchful waiting" approach to keep an eye on it, a diet low in meat and eggs is a very good idea.

Reluctant to give up animal products? Then think about this: In a study where prostate cancer patients were asked to eat a plant-based diet, nine of the ten patients experienced a slowing of their PSA growth rate and four of them experienced an actual reversal in their PSA levels and cancer growth.

If you want to live a long, comfortable life, then it's worth getting on board. Food that makes you happier, healthier, and is NOT socially limiting. One final note: It's not just cancer and depression that respond to lower levels of arachidonic acid. Chronic health issues like inflammatory bowel disease, including ulcerative colitis and Crohn's disease, get better when people consume lower levels of arachidonic acid. This is achieved by eliminating animal protein from the diet. Basically, skip the mea and eggs. (Note: Even a semi-vegetarian diet seems to help with Crohn's patients.) There's more: patients with rheumatoid arthritis seem to improve on vegetarian diets, and it's possible they're benefiting from the anti-inflammatory effects of lower levels of arachidonic acid.

The change in eating habits may not be as hard as you think. In one study that put patients on a strict vegetarian diet, the researchers were initially worried that participants would find the diet hard and socially limiting. They even thought it might lead to psychological distress. On the contrary, their patients scored higher than ever in their measures of psychological health and reported less depression and anxiety.

So limit those eggs. They may be delicious but remember: We eat to live, not live to eat.

Health benefits of lycopene and cabbage

Researchers have found that lycopene, the carotenoid pigment that gives tomatoes and watermelons much of their red hue, may soon be recognized as an important weapon against cancer. Lycopene is one of the most powerful antioxidants you can consume -- but not in the form in which it is found in tomatoes, watermelon and other produce.

You see, the relatively large molecules that compose lycopene in your vegetables and fruits are constructed in microscopic straight lines. These are referred to as trans-isomers (Isomers are the various, different geometric constructions of the atoms that make up the molecules in chemicals.)

According to researchers, the form of lycopene that can most effectively zap free radicals in the human body is in a more rounded configuration – what are known as cis-isomers. How the straight isomers become the rounded types used by the body has puzzled researchers. But studies now indicate that the digestive system takes the straight-line lycopene you swallow in food and converts it to the rounded, more beneficial form with the help of stomach acid.

However, researchers also believe that if the acidity of your stomach is too low, the conversion of lycopene to its more powerful antioxidant form may not be very efficient – another reason not to take medications that reduce your stomach acid.

Clobbers free radicals

Studies of the antioxidant powers of lycopene in the body have produced astounding results. Consider how lycopene can deal with what is known as singlet oxygen, a particularly harmful oxidative free radical that can injure cell membranes, distort genetic material and oxidize amino acids (protein building blocks).

While many other antioxidants can vanquish only a few free radical molecules at a time and then have to be restored to their original state before performing more antioxidant tasks, scientists have shown one molecule of lycopene can disarm about 1,000 molecules of singlet oxygen.2 The reason is that lycopene rebounds back to its active form almost instantly after disarming a free radical. This ability makes it the single most effective antioxidant among all the carotenoids found in plants.

Support group for glutathione and SOD

Aside from its role as an antioxidant, lycopene also spurs the body to ramp up its production of its own antioxidant defenses that can keep cells and their structures from being damaged. As researchers put it, lycopene "upregulates" the body's "antioxidant response element."

What they mean is that with the help of lycopene the cells produce more cellular enzymes like superoxide dismutase (SOD), quinone reductase and glutathione S-transferase which can all fend off attack by free radicals. (In technical terms, these are known as "cytoprotective" enzymes.) Scientists know that superoxide dismutase and glutathione are enormously powerful antioxidants that our own bodies make – especially if we give the body the nutrition it needs.

Activating an activator

These protective enzymes result from lycopene stimulating a protein called NRF2, which constantly travels in out of a cell's nucleus (where the genetic material is contained) and in and out of the cell to keep track of a cell's health and how it is functioning. Of all the carotenoids found in plants, lycopene has been shown to be the most active in increasing levels of Nrf2.

When a cell is confronted with toxins, free radicals or some other circumstance that threatens its well-being, NRF2 speeds up its activity, moving more quickly, and starts calling for the cell to accelerate its production of antioxidants.

According to research at the University of Warwick Medical School, in England, it is not only toxins or an oxidative threat that leads NRF2 to speed up its movement. While NRF2 usually takes more than two hours to move in and out of a cell, a substance like lycopene cuts this cycle time down to about 80 minutes, boosting NRF2's ability to survey the cell's micro-environment. "The way NRF2 works is very similar to sensors in electronic devices that rely on continual reassessment of their surroundings to provide an appropriate response," says researcher Paul Thornalley.

Attacking cancer's energy source

Aside from these roles in the body, lycopene has now also been shown to eradicate cancer cells by degrading their mitochondria, thereby leading the cells to undergo apoptosis – their own programmed cell death. In a study of prostate cancer cells, researchers found that, on the first exposure to lycopene, the mitochondria in the cells start to have trouble functioning. Then their membranes became leaky, releasing proteins from the mitochondria into the cell's protoplasm. Once those proteins began to stream through the mitochondrial membranes, elimination of the cells via apoptosis was not far behind.

In addition, other research shows that lycopene can reduce cancer cells' production of integrins, chemicals they need in order to proliferate in the body, stick to tissues and invade organs. The loss of integrins can make tumors less aggressive, less likely to metastasize and slower to spread.

Less risk of cancer, and younger skin to boot

All of these effects of lycopene are probably the reason that a study in England shows that men who eat ten or more helpings of tomatoes a week enjoy an 18 percent lower risk of prostate cancer. The study compared the lifestyle habits and diets of more than 1,800 men aged 50 to 69 who had prostate cancer with more than 12,000 men who were cancer-free.

"Our findings suggest that tomatoes may be important in prostate cancer prevention," says researcher Vanessa Er. Of course, as most researchers do, she still hedges her bets: "However, further studies need to be conducted to confirm our findings, especially through human trials," she adds. "Men should still eat a wide variety of fruits and vegetables, maintain a healthy weight and stay active."

Even if it weren't so great at helping protect your body against cancer, you should get plenty of this nutrient to help your skin and face stay better looking. Research in Germany shows that lycopene helps defend the skin against sun damage and could even keep you from getting wrinkled.

A potent cancer fighter

Cabbage doesn't get the fanfare other vegetables do. But it should. Especially if it's red cabbage. Cabbage contains many potent anti-cancer substances. One that stands above the rest is glucosinolates that break down into indoles, sulforaphane, and other cancer-preventive substances.

The glucosinolates of cabbage convert to isothiocyanate compounds. These, in turn, prevent many cancers – including cancers of the bladder, breast, colon, and prostate. Your cell cycle is a rigidly controlled set of steps your cells undergo before they divide into two. Before that final split, a cell must duplicate all its contents, so the two daughter cells are exact clones of the parent.

This means if you can alter specific components of the cell's cycle, you can keep cancer cells from growing, without killing normal cells. Sulforaphane – another by-product of glucosinolates – selectively targets cancer stem cells, thereby helping to keep cancer in check.

Certain compounds in cabbage change how your body uses estrogen, which may prevent breast cancer. Cabbage also boasts powerful antioxidants and anti-inflammatory benefits. Researchers have linked H. pylori with stomach cancer. Back in the 1800s, cancer surgeons thought stomach cancer was linked to ulcers, citing inflammation and persistent stomach irritation. But no one really understood it. To make matters worse, before the 1980s, dominant dogma attributed ulcers and gastritis to stress and diet.

That changed in the early 1980s when two Australian scientists noticed that most ulcer patients had H. pylori bacteria. Their claims were dismissed amid the belief that bacteria couldn't possibly survive in stomach acid. To prove his point one of the scientists, Barry Marshall, heroically drank a broth containing H. pylori. Sure enough, he quickly got gastritis. Fortunately, that was before antibiotic resistance had become widespread, so he was able to cure himself of his self-induced illness with antibiotics. Today, it's widely accepted that H. pylori triggers ulcers and chronic gastritis.

Chinese study reveals a secret link

Meanwhile, other researchers tried to tease out stomach cancer triggers. In the 1970s, a large South American study showed that long-term stomach inflammation is often associated with stomach cancer. A link, but still no proof of how one caused the other.

But scientists also knew that stomach cancer rates were highest in infection-prone areas. Finally a 1990 study collected blood samples from Chinese men of all ages living where H. pylori infections were rampant... then matched them to death records. The results were shocking. Stomach cancer deaths were the only cancer deaths related to H. pylori infection.

Today stomach cancer is the second biggest cancer killer worldwide. If you have H. pylori infection, you're a whopping six times more likely to develop stomach cancer than if you don't. Cabbage juice contains a huge amount of vitamin U. Technically it's not a vitamin... it's an enzyme called S-methylmethionine and sometimes dubbed "cabbagen."

Vitamin U effectively promotes rapid healing of peptic ulcers. Cabbage also stimulates your stomach to produce acid. And while you might not think that's a good thing, it is. Many people have low stomach acid, which it turns out is a hidden cause of digestive issues. Low stomach acid drastically boosts your risk of infections. So enjoying a few teaspoons of cabbage juice (or better yet, fermented cabbage juice from sauerkraut) before meals can do wonders for your digestion.

Red cabbage or green cabbage?

Not all cabbage is the same. Red cabbage isn't the same as green. And it's not just about looks. It's about nutritional profile. To be clear, no matter what color cabbage you eat, you can hardly go wrong. They're both low in calories, high in fiber and nutrients. Cabbage is ranked fifth on the Environmental Working Group's list of the "Clean 15" veggies, containing less pesticide residue than other produce. As vegetables go, cabbage is also pretty inexpensive. But make note of these differences between red and green.

Red cabbage – or purple or blue depending on soil pH – contains ten times more vitamin A than green cabbage. One cup of chopped red cabbage provides a third of your recommended daily intake of vitamin A. An equal amount of green cabbage only gives three percent. Vitamin A helps prevent early stage macular degeneration from progressing to blindness. It promotes healthy teeth, skin, tissues, and immune system.

One cup of chopped red cabbage has 51 milligrams of Vitamin C, whereas green cabbage only contains 37 milligrams. Anti-inflammatory nutrients called anthocyanins are only found in red cabbage. They give it the red or purple color. Besides their anti-cancer benefits, these nutrients help improve memory and promote weight loss.

Iron carries oxygen to your cells for energy and DNA synthesis. Your immune system needs it to fight viruses. Most of us don't need more iron (you should not take iron supplements, for example, unless a blood test shows you need them.) But you do need some iron, and if you don't eat red meat you need to find vegetable sources for the mineral.

Red cabbage has twice the iron of green cabbage. But green cabbage outshines red cabbage for vitamin K (for blood clotting and bone density). One cup of chopped green cabbage provides 57 percent of your daily requirements, compared to just 28 percent in red cabbage. Low vitamin K equates to increased risk of hip fracture.

Best ways to prepare cabbage

To get the most from your cabbage, eat it raw or barely cooked (tender-crisp). Otherwise you'll lose its anti-cancer effects. All cooking methods reduce anthocyanins, glucosinolates and other nutrients. And skip the microwave. It destroys cancer-fighting enzymes.

Cabbage is popular as a primary fermented vegetable. Sauerkraut is an excellent choice, and try to get it unpasteurized, because it will then be rich in probiotics.

Other do's and don'ts:

• Use firm, undamaged, unblemished heads of cabbage. No limp leaves.

• Buy the whole head – not pre-cut or shredded, as the processing loses nutrients to oxidation.

• Drink your cabbage juice fresh. Don't refrigerate.

• Limit yourself to four ounces of cabbage juice at once. Best, drink small amounts three times a day on an empty stomach.

• If you have a thyroid disorder, avoid large quantities of cabbage. It can interfere with iodine absorption.

• Rotate the various types of cabbage into your diet for broadest health benefits.

• Cabbage may trigger gassiness in some people.

Quick super salad recipe:

For a tasty cabbage superfood salad, mix shredded cabbage, chopped kale, carrots, golden beets, orange slices, green onions, Goji berries, raw cashews, sunflower seeds, orange juice, one to two teaspoons sesame oil, sea salt and sesame seeds for garnish.

Cheap nano medicine - the third prong

It's "a disgrace...a cruel deception....nonsense on stilts....witchcraft" says Dr Tom Dolphin, deputy chair of the British Medical Association's junior doctors committee. He's angry and he's not alone. What makes him so mad? Why, it's just another exciting alternative treatment breakthrough.

Dr. Dolphin's disgust is shared by many of his colleagues concerning this 200-year-old form of medicine - or quackery as they see it. They say it has no place in a modern medical system. They believe something so "scientifically implausible" should not be available as part of the UK's National Health Service – which allows doctors to prescribe it for a wide range of health conditions, including the side effects of radiation and chemotherapy.

Not only is it used as supportive therapy for cancer, but in some places outside the UK it's prescribed – amazing to say -- as a front line therapy and even as the sole therapy for cancer. This happens in a clinic in India where the Banerji Protocols, a modern version of an 18th century medical system started by Dr Samuel Hahnemann, are used to treat over a hundred cancer patients a day. The doctors who run the clinic achieve some astonishing results.

The therapy I'm talking about is homeopathy.

Classical homeopathy vs the Banerji Protocols

Homeopathy contends that a substance that causes a particular set of symptoms when taken in a large dose by a healthy person can be used to treat the same symptoms when taken in a tiny dose. This is the like-cures-like principle.

An example might be a plant that causes your skin to itch. Taken in an extremely small dose diluted in water, an extract of this plant may cure itching skin.

Homeopathic medicines may be derived from plants, animal products or minerals. They are diluted and succussed (shaken) until the desired dosage is achieved. The more the substance is diluted the stronger the remedy is said to become.

A remedy can get diluted to the point where almost nothing is left of the original source material. This aspect is what creates such incredulity among "proper" scientifically-trained doctors. I have to admit it sounds like quackery. But there is published research by medical doctors which suggests it can be effective.

In traditional or classical homeopathy developed by the German doctor Samuel Hahnemann in the late 1700s, a single dose of a single medicine is given to the patient based on the person's symptoms and individual constitution. Different remedies may be used for two different patients who have the same disease, because the choice of medicine is not based just on the disease but on the whole patient, seen in his or her entirety as an individual.

So many people came to see the first Dr. Pareshnath Banerji when he started his clinic in 1918 that he wasn't able to spend the amount of time needed to get to know the person in a traditional homeopathic consultation. So he would prescribe the same remedy or even a combination of remedies to patients for common conditions, and despite this departure from the ideal approach, he reportedly saw a high rate of success.

The tradition continues today with Prasanta Banerji and his son Pratip at their clinic in Kolkata, who use a more objective approach than in traditional homeopathy. They utilize advanced tests and tools such as magnetic resonance imaging (MRI) and ultrasound images for diagnosis.

And they've used their considerable experience to prescribe particular medicines in specific potencies and in fixed dosages for cancer and other diseases. This standardized strategy – as opposed to the individualized approach -- makes it easy to learn, easy to apply and should give more reproducible results.

The National Cancer Institute finds evidence of possible efficacy

The doctors Banerji began testing homeopathy for cancer patients in 1992. Later in the decade they gave a six hour presentation on 16 cases of brain tumor regression before oncologists from leading American cancer centers at an international conference.

The National Institutes of Health (NIH) asked them to submit records of successful cases for their Best Case program. This allows practitioners outside conventional medicine to present data for appraisal. After detailed evaluation by the National Cancer Institute (NCI), four cases were accepted for publication in the journal Oncology Reports in 2008. Two of these patients presented with cancers of the esophagus and two with lung cancer. All four became symptom free and enjoyed highly positive outcomes. None of them received any conventional treatment. The NCI found the results were sufficient to warrant further research.

Encouraging results at MD Anderson

Several studies were carried out by the Banerjis in conjunction with the M.D. Anderson Cancer Center in Houston. In the first study, researchers tested two homeopathic remedies, Ruta 6 in combination with calcium phosphate, on normal cells and brain cancer cells. This study also included 15 case reports of patients with brain tumors treated at Kolkata. The patients were 10 to 65 years of age and were mostly at an advanced stage. They were treated for up to seven years with the same two remedies. They received neither chemotherapy nor radiation.

In both the lab work and in patients "results showed induction of survival-signaling pathways in normal lymphocytes and induction of death signaling pathways in brain cancer cells." Out of the seven patients suffering from glioma, a type of brain cancer, six "showed complete regression of tumors." The authors concluded that the remedies "could be used for effective treatment of brain cancers, particularly glioma.

Dr. Moshe Frenkel from M.D. Anderson helped arrange the study. He was so impressed, he traveled to India to visit the Banerji clinic in person. "I saw things there that I couldn't explain. Tumors shrank with nothing else other than homeopathic remedies...X-rays showing there is a lesion on the lung and a year after taking the remedy it has shrunk or disappeared."

Dr Frankel, together with seven of his colleagues, carried out a second laboratory study which tested four homeopathic remedies on breast cancer cells. "The remedies exerted preferential cytotoxic effects...causing cell cycle delay/arrest and apoptosis [cancer cell death]." They even found that two of the remedies were similar in their effects to the activity of Taxol, a chemotherapy drug commonly prescribed for breast cancer.

Also impressed was Barbara Sarter, Ph.D., Associate Professor in Advanced Practice Nursing at the University of San Diego, who also travelled to India. "For the most aggressive and lethal of brain tumors they are able to cure one out of three patients, compared to the five percent cure rate with conventional treatments of surgery, chemotherapy and radiation," she said.

According to the Banerjis' own data, between 1990 and 2005 they treated 21,888 patients for malignant tumors. Although these patients did not undergo any conventional treatment, there was complete regression in 19% and tumors were static or improved in 21%.

Critics will point to the fact that all the evidence the Banerjis have ever presented at conferences or in published studies is observational in a small number of patients. Until high quality studies are carried out the Banerji Protocols will never be accepted by conventional medicine.

Such studies are unlikely to ever take place. But even if they did, the lack of a plausible mechanism for how homeopathy works makes it likely that many orthodox doctors would still reject it. For one thing a double blind study cannot be undertaken on a protocol where the dose of medicine is barely perceptible. Yet it appears to work.

Homeopathy as a form of nanomedicine

Many researchers into homeopathy believe it works by hormesis, whereby a substance that is toxic in a large dose can have the reverse effect -- be stimulatory or beneficial -- in a small dose. This is an accepted concept in pharmacology and toxicology. A tiny dose can act as a mild stressor which sets off an adaptive response throughout the whole body.

But no stressor (hormetin) appears to be visible in a

typical homeopathic remedy because of the high dilutions.

This changed in 2010. Using sophisticated electron microscopes, original source materials were found in highly diluted homeopathic remedies as nanoparticles. Nanoparticles are very potent because of their highly charged properties and multiple effects. They can enter cells easily because of their small size -- similar to a virus -- and be precisely targeted. Nanostructured forms of drugs are a growing segment of conventional medicine.

There are many possibilities for this form of medical nanotechnology, such as delivering nanoparticles to a cell to instruct it to behave in a different way -- like an intelligent molecular-scale mechanic working on damaged cells. Homeopathic remedies work as nanomedicines, according to the Banerjis and colleagues from three centers in the United State, writing in a recent research paper.

They say, "In one sense, homeopaths in clinical practice may be many years ahead of conventional physicians in applied understanding of how and when to use nanoparticles of natural products for safe and effective clinical treatment."

Prong Three of the Cornish Protocol

Homeopathy was the third spear thrust at the heart of my prostate cancer treatment, and covers the other important 50% of beating cancer as I explained earlier in the book. The three remedies I used with food and exercise effectively caused my tumor to reduce and eventually disappear. To this day I no longer fear cancer because of these remedies. For I know I can go back to them again if it ever returns and achieve the same results, again and again and again.

In my case I used three remedies, the last one (Rhus Tox 6C) added to the known remedies for prostate cancer(Sabal Serrulata (Saw palmetto) and a common remedy that will help diminish almost any other cancer - Thuja Occidentalis.

If you were expecting me to talk of the new immunology treatments here, you are mistaken. There is no reference to experimental methods still being tested today in labs or radical prostatectomy or new chemotherapy drugs or anything of that sort. But this area is highly controversial because few people understand how it works. I am talking of homeopathy remedies.

Having practiced homeopathy for over 10 years, I am now in a position to tell you that I have used this medicine successfully to treat my own cancer, sending it to into full diminishment and eventual disappearance. I am not talking "remission" here but completely gone, nada, zip. With no side effects, with nary any pain or discomfort and most importantly with no effect on my Mojo. And that last point I think most men can identify with. My PSA levels at its peak were at 6.1 and now stand at a mere 1.2, well within the safe range of 0-2. The tumor mass of 1 cm is shrunk to a point where it is now no longer visible. I expect that 5 years into the future, should I stick to my healthy diet, I should NOT see it recur. With surgical incision or chemotherapy, the body gets weaker especially if you are older, and there is an 80% chance of remission after 5 years. This method eliminates it entirely, whenever you need it. If you slack off on your diet or feel that you are becoming unhealthy again, all you need to do is get back to healthy eating, rinse and repeat what is covered in this chapter.

NOTE: Homeopathy does not lend itself to double blind testing. For one the same remedy does not have the same effect on everyone. One remedy will be the right one for 30-50% of people and another one may be needed to address the same condition in another 30-50% of patents. Thuja Occidentals on the other hand is a common remedy I would propose as a starting point to diminish all kinds of cancers. As I mentioned before, homeopathic "medicine" would not pass a double blind trial against a medicine whose dosage and active ingredient range is much much higher than a homeopathy remedy, at least 100,000 to 1 million times more active dosage.

So you may ask - how in the deuce does homeopathy work ?

The way homeopathy works is not by brute force but by a gentle shift or triggering of the body's OWN immune system. The amount of active substance though small is sufficient in small dose of 30C (the scale will be explained below) to shift the body into fighting symptoms induced externally by the remedy, which just happen to be symptoms of prostate disease. The situation is akin to warning the body of a bigger enemy it needs to fight by pointing to a smaller one that has the same effect. Hope this helps understand how it works - essentially a homeopathic remedy triggers the body to act against something smaller (the remedy which is typically a toxin that is harmless in nanoparticles), and redirect the body's immune system to engulf the larger problem while it's doing that.

My treatment of my cancer started with the homeopathy remedy Sabal Serrulata. Most of you may recognize this as the latin name of Saw Palmetto, a well known supplement taken for BPH or benign prostate hyperplasia. The same substance when homeopathized is even more powerful than increased dosages of that supplement. Trust me, it works even better! Starting with Sabal Serrul. 30C every 3 days to a week, I began to see improvement in my enuresis symptoms at night and control over the bladder. A second remedy to target the bladder is made from American Arborvitae (latin name - Thuja occidentalis). This is also taken in 30C dosage of the remedy. These remedies were from the Boiron brand, which is readily available and cheap to boot, coming in at about 60-70 pellets per $8 tube. You only need 3 - 5 pellets under the tongue once per 2-3 days treatment, giving you a 3-month supply at $8! I told you I was cheap !

Thuja Occidentalis contains the poison absinthe which was used a a drink by philosophers two centuries ago because it induced "clarity of the mind". And a final remedy I added to the two that worked was specifically tailored to my own disposition. This was Rhus Toxicodendron. With this trio of remedies I began on the road to recovery after incorporating the first two prongs of healthy mindful anti-inflammatory eating and moderate exercise. Within days the effects were clearly visible. While anti-inflammatory eating took up the first 30% of my recovery and exercise another 20%, it is the last 50% that put me firmly on the road to a complete and lasting cure. Hence my three-pronged strategy.

By no means should you think that I am against conventional medicine along with methods used such as surgical incision, radial prostatectomy, chemotherapy or radiation. These methods will address your tumor to the point where it is removed and rendered relatively harmless but only for a short period of a few years at most. The source of such radial sickness still radiates from the point where it was found, namely the prostate and the risk of relapse will remain high. Whether that happens in 5 or 10 years or even less than five years depends on how aggressive the cancer is. Your survivability depends on how aggressive the inflammation is. If it is fairly aggressive, you are looking at more of the same invasive treatment down the road at an older, more vulnerable age when your immune system is further weakened. On the other hand, you could use these homeopathy remedies as an adjunct treatment set up entirely by yourself to start, stop or to alleviate the inflammation at the same site.

The best part of homeopathy is that it directs itself to trigger the body to correct its own immune response to the inflammation. After the trigger is set by the remedy - typically 3-4 tiny pellets placed under the tongue, the body begins to work towards remedying the inflammation. You could start with Sabal Serrulata 30C. At this point you should make notes or journal. If you have BPH and night enuresis, you will slowly start to see a drop in the need to urinate several times at night. You may also be pleasantly surprised to see a regrowth of hair(if you are losing hair) at the crown of your head. I call this a pleasant side effect of Sabal Serrulata. It works by not allowing the conversion of testosterone to di-hydrotestosterone which is involved both in increasing conditions of BPH and loss of hair especially so visible on the crown. It is not however a cure for alopecia or hereditary baldness!

Some of you have seen the youtube video where Richard Dawkins tries to debunk homeopathy by going to the ocean and dropping a test-tube of liquid into the water and telling the viewers that expecting the medication to work after he had poured it in and retrieved a test-tube of the water from the ocean would be laughable. And indeed it would be, with an open ended ocean. Well, I have news for you - that isn't a very good analogy. There are better equivalent scenarios to draw from to understand the power of gentle homeopathy. For one thing homeopathy even in liquid form is a closed system, not where you pour something in and retrieve something out. There is the process of succession that increases the strength of the remedy. You can skip liquid remedies however as I did it, and simply stick to dry pellets of 30C dosage, taken every 2-3 days or so.

If you still doubt homeopathy really works, I have a simple anecdote for you. Dr Noam Sobel who's an international expert on the olfactory(sense of smell) system from the University of Berkeley, once offered an interesting take of the human ability to smell. He said if you took two Olympic size swimming pools and dropped just 1 ml of a deodorant into one pool, you could tell the difference between the pools just from your sense of smell. Unbelievable? This would however be a better analogy to how homeopathy works. The body can sense minute amounts of a substance in a greater quantity of substrate or base liquid like water in ways we can't even imagine.

When I felt a tiny stabbing pain in the bladder, I would take Sabal Serrulata 30C. If I had more than the usual urination frequency, I would supplement with Rhus Tox 6C and sometimes with Thuja Occidentalis 30C. This is where you take notes at least at the beginning. You will know when to select Rhus Tox 6C or Thuja Occidentals 30C or both together if needed every 2-3 days. In my case unnatural urination frequency dropped within months to the point where I was more comfortable till the present day where I operate normally without worrying about imbibing liquids before I go to bed.

Suffice it to say, I was sold on this cheap and effective mode of treatment. With no dependence on the medical system through COVID, I was a happy camper. My health improved every day till I no longer worried about my prostate on a daily basis. Now-a-days it hardly crosses my mind.

Other forms of cancer

While I did not use the Banerji protocol for prostate cancer and stuck to my own researched treatment using the Materia Medica of homeopathy, you will notice some similarity at least with our common use of Thuja Occidentalis which I consider an all weather important remedy for cancer and the universal use of Sabal Serrulata (saw palmetto) for the prostate. If you suffer from other forms of cancer, I would Google their free link for remedies they commonly use since I do not have personal experience in those forms of cancer. You might be pleasantly surprised at what you can achieve yourselves with limited resources.

For example for Breast cancer, they suggest the remedy Phytolacca (decandra) 200C (Pokeweed) and in the third stage they employ Thuja Occidentalis again. For Rectal cancer, they once again use Thuja Occidentalis in the third stage (I would imply it sooner as a first remedy instead). For colon cancer, they may suggest Hydrastis(cannadensis) or Goldenseal as a first remedy. I would also experiment using Thuja Occidentalis in all these forms as a common remedy. This one's a personal favorite so I cannot repeat it enough.

You can easily get these remedies in the Boiron brand. Personally I prefer the Boiron or Reckeweg brands, rather than use unknown brands of questionable quality. Even the infrequent use of Thuja Occidentalis and its effects can provide much needed relief to a long sufferer. Of course none of these will help unless you also implement the first two preliminary steps of reducing or eliminating pro-inflammatory foods and partake in some daily exercise to get the lymphatic system moving to further detoxify your body. These have been covered in other chapters in this book.

Artificial sweeteners or embalmers

You may love seeing 'zero calories' on your favorite beverages. But the sweetener that makes them 'zero calorie' is poisonous. And it makes cancer grow like wildfire. Wildfires take no prisoners. They ruthlessly destroy everything in their path. So why would you do anything that makes cancer grow like wildfire?

To take just the most common sweetener, no sooner do you gulp or slurp down an aspartame-sweetened beverage than your body breaks it down into formaldehyde and other cancer-causing toxins. Formaldehyde is an embalming fluid. It's also used as a paint remover.

And aspartame is not just in beverages. The food industry loves this substance and uses it pervasively – to the tune of 6,000 food products. Aspartame is added liberally to diet soda, chewing gum, frozen and packaged desserts, yogurt, chewable vitamins, and many things you wouldn't suspect are in need of sweetening.

Nor is it just aspartame. The FDA has approved many different artificial sweeteners, and we can't possibly cover all of them in detail in this report. I think these sweeteners taste terrible. Obviously, other people disagree and think they taste good, but these chemicals do severe health damage.

Animal studies suggest these sweeteners can be very addictive – even more so than cocaine. A study of rats showed that, given a choice between cocaine or saccharin, most of the rats chose saccharin. Now can you see why this substance is added to so many foods?

More good reasons not to eat foods that turn into formaldehyde

Aspartame — sold under the brand names NutraSweet and Equal — is 200 times sweeter than sugar. The chemical is made up of three main ingredients: phenylalanine, aspartic acid, and methanol. In nature, methanol binds to the fiber pectin, allowing it to pass through your body safely. But methanol as it's found in aspartame (without fiber) binds to amino acids and converts to formaldehyde. Formaldehyde causes serious DNA damage leading to cancer – especially breast and prostate cancers, which have risen in sync with increasing aspartame use.

Dr. Russell Blaylock, retired neurosurgeon and author of Excitotoxins: The Taste That Kills, says that drinking just one diet soda a day causes formaldehyde buildup in your cells... which accumulates day after day. That kind of compounding will kill you.

Throws your brain cells into a frenzy

Aspartic acid — another aspartame ingredient — literally excites your brain cells to death. The official term is excitotoxicity. This means aspartic acid stimulates ('excites') your neurons and nerve cells until they die. Monosodium glutamate (MSG) works similarly.

Aspartic acid (and MSG) 'pokes' holes in your brain where these overactive brain cells die. Excitotoxins also produce free radicals that damage your tissues and organs, causing arthritis, cardiovascular disease, and cancer.

Just two years after aspartame first appeared in diet sodas, brain cancer increased ten percent, according to the National Cancer Institute. A causal connection hasn't been proved, but it seems probable. When aspartic acid hits cancer cells, they immediately start multiplying faster.

Cancer cells are a normal phenomenon – we all have them. It's when they multiply faster than our immune system can kill them that we get in trouble. A substance that speeds up the multiplication of rogue cells is the perfect fuel for cancer.

Dr. Blaylock says excitotoxins make cancer cells 'grow like wildfire.' And if you've tried everything you know to lose weight and just can't seem to succeed, maybe it's because of this - your brain is tricked into eating too much. Ironically, instead of helping you lose weight, artificial sweeteners boost your risk of diabetes and obesity, which are also linked to cancer (diabetes doubles the risk of some kinds of cancer). A 14-year study of 66,118 women showed that drinking a single 12-ounce diet soda per day increased their risk of type-2 diabetes by one-third. With a 20-ounce diet soda, the diabetes risk doubled.

Diet soda also increased their risk of obesity 200 percent. To put it in plain English, diet sodas make you fat. You see, when you eat something sweet, your brain releases a chemical called dopamine that triggers your brain's reward center. Then once you eat a certain number of calories, a hormone called leptin signals your brain that you're full.

But artificial sweeteners confuse those signals and induce

cravings because you haven't eaten those calories. When you eat something that tastes sweet but has no calories (i.e., artificial sweeteners), dopamine triggers your brain. But leptin never shuts it off. So, artificial sweeteners actually breed intense sugar cravings and overeating. When you eat or drink anything 'zero-calorie,' you escalate hunger and cravings. I'll say it again: Diet sodas make you fat. I can't think of any reason at all to eat a "diet" food that actually makes you fat, and causes diabetes and cancer to boot. And tastes bad.

As mentioned, many foods contain artificial sweeteners (and many others contain sugar, including the food industry's favorite form of sugar, high fructose corn syrup). So health begins with learning to read labels (I speak from experience). So many processed foods contain either aspartame or sugar, you will find yourself not eating most of them. The best policy is to totally give up processed and manufactured foods. Eat fresh ingredients – fruits and vegetables (organic if at all possible, to avoid chemicals).

If you're looking for a halfway house, don't eat processed foods that contain more than four or five ingredients. When the list of ingredients is so long it runs off the end of the page – and you've never heard of most of them -- then eating that food is probably a bad idea.

Weedkiller in your food

I'm sure that none of us, if we had the choice, would voluntarily swallow a toxin that increases the risk of cancer. But in the real world, our daily choices aren't so clear cut. Our world is saturated in chemicals, and you can't avoid them all. You have to choose your battles.

Glyphosate is in the news lately because a California court awarded $289 million in damages to a man who says the herbicide caused his cancer. He frequently handled the chemical as part of his job as a groundskeeper, so his exposure was probably much higher than you and I would ever ingest in food.

The case is on appeal, and meanwhile thousands of other lawsuits are pending. Originally glyphosate was only available under the brand name Roundup, but the patent has expired, and now many different companies market the chemical under different names. Under any name, it's long been a target of activist groups.

Huge amounts in farm fields across the US

There are plenty of less harmful methods farmers can implement that would control weeds while using less glyphosate. We need to be more prudent about how much of it we use, but at the same time I don't think we need to panic and ban it altogether.

In the eyes of many critics, the worst thing about glyphosate is that it goes hand in hand with genetically modified crops. These crops are engineered to survive being sprayed with glyphosate, so the net result is that the herbicide just kills the weeds while it spares the crops.

How much does glyphosate add to a person's risk of cancer? According to Arthur Lambert, a researcher at the Whitehead Institute of Biomedical Research in Cambridge, Massachusetts, "even if one accepts the high end of the reported risks (for cancer) the effects (of glyphosate) are, at best, modest." As Dr. Lambert points out, while smoking increases your cancer risk by up to 2,000 percent (i.e. by a factor of 20), the highest estimate of glyphosate's increased risk from exposure is about 30 percent.

Amounts being consumed have soared

It's hard to estimate the impact of glyphosate on cancer risk for many reasons. One of them is that our national use of this toxin has been increasing. Researchers at the University of California San Diego School of Medicine have found that since farmers began growing genetically modified (GMO) foods in the 1990s, human exposure to glyphosate – from food residues – has gone up on average by around 500 percent.

Because cancer takes decades to develop, in most cases, we haven't yet seen the impact on cancer rates that may result from the recent, massive increase in consumption. The California scientists have measured levels of glyphosates by analyzing chemicals excreted in people's urine since 1993 when farmers first started raising GMO crops. Many GMO crops that are now in our food have been genetically modified to survive the glyphosate exposure that kills weeds.

"Our exposure to these chemicals has increased significantly over the years but most people are unaware that they are consuming them through their diet," warns researcher Paul J. Mills. "What we saw (in our research) was that prior to the introduction of genetically modified foods, very few people had detectable levels of glyphosate," says Dr. Mills.

Now, however, 70 percent of us have the chemical in our bodies, he warns. He adds that use of the herbicide has gone up about 15-fold during the past 25 years, because farmers have increasingly planted the GMO crops designed to survive being sprayed. Glyphosate is applied most often to GMO soy and corn, but it's also applied to wheat and oats grown in the US.

Inactive ingredients – or not?

Researchers have also focused on questions about how herbicides are formulated: The other chemicals that are mixed into glyphosate-based herbicides can also affect health. Although glyphosate is allegedly the only "active" ingredient in many herbicide products, researchers in England point out that the "adjuvant" ingredients that are combined with glyphosate, and which are considered "inactive," can pose health difficulties that get overlooked when herbicides and pesticides are studied for their physiological effects.

"Exposure to environmental levels of some of these adjuvant mixtures can affect non-target organisms -- and even can cause chronic human disease," warns researcher Robin Mesnage of King's College London. "Despite this, adjuvants are not currently subject to an acceptable daily intake and are not included in the health risk assessment of dietary exposures to pesticide residues."

Another concern: Studies show that an increased cancer

risk isn't the only health issue linked to glyphosate. For example, researchers at the University of California – San Diego have also found the herbicide may be linked to liver problems.4 When they looked at people suffering what's called nonalcoholic fatty liver disease (NAFLD), it turned out that their levels of glyphosate were significantly higher than in people with healthy livers.

And, these California researchers note, lab studies have similarly indicated that glyphosate can give your liver a hard time. "There have been a handful of studies, all of which we cited in our paper, where animals either were or weren't fed Roundup or glyphosate directly, and they all point to the same thing: the development of liver pathology," says Dr. Mills.

Problems can be passed down to children

Meanwhile, tests at Washington State University raise the possibility that health issues caused by glyphosate may be inter-generational – your exposure to glyphosate may affect your children and grandchildren. These lab studies, done on rodents, found that glyphosate exposure during pregnancy may cause prostate, kidney and ovarian problems in offspring and later generations. They also found the herbicide is statistically linked to a bigger risk of being obese and suffering birth abnormalities.

The researchers conclude that we need to take the risk to future generations into account when analyzing the safety of glyphosate and other toxins. "The ability of glyphosate and other environmental toxicants to impact our future generations needs to be considered and is potentially as important as the direct exposure toxicology done today for risk assessment."

Eat organic when possible

Try to eat organic food whenever possible but don't obsess about it. Some exposure to low levels of a chemical like glyphosate may not be a significant factor in your health. And in light of how our food supply is grown and produced, some exposure to glyphosate is probably unavoidable, anyway.

Cancer has many, many possible causes, and most of us have been exposed to a large number of them. Probably each and every one of us has been exposed to dozens of deadly toxins. For most of these toxins, the exposure has to be pretty high, and last for a long time, to "cause" someone's cancer. And even then the cancer will likely take decades to develop. So if you have cancer it's next to impossible to put your finger on one cause and say, "This is it, this is what gave me cancer."

Little is known about the interactions among all the different causes of cancer. For example, it's known that the combination of asbestos exposure AND a smoking habit is lethal. Studies likewise suggest that drinking alcohol regularly PLUS smoking is much more risky than either one by itself. But in general we don't know much about the lethal synergies of all these carcinogens.

That doesn't mean we should carelessly accept glyphosate in our food. We need systemic changes to our agricultural system to bring the use of glyphosate and other pesticides down. It's also clear the regulatory authorities are worse than useless at identifying carcinogens and denying corporations the right to put them in products. In that sense, the folks who campaign against glyphosate – and other activists who wage war against other toxins – are doing good work. So try to eat organic when possible but don't obsess. That's it.

5G EMF, prostate cancer and plunging sperm counts

Wireless devices of all kinds – cell phones, cell towers, tablets, Alexa, the wireless router in your home, the WiFi hotspots that are almost everywhere – pose a deadly danger to health. Among the worst dangers (admittedly not confirmed yet) is that they cause infertility and are responsible for plunging birth rates in those places that are most densely networked. It is possible that, within a few years, hundreds of millions of people will be unable to have children and whole societies may dwindle to nothing.

The wireless industry is so vast it has, in a sense, become the whole economy. It's the entire high tech industry and all the myriad industries from cars to utility meters that are now wired. All of us depend on devices that emit or receive EMFs, and it's hard to imagine life without them.

As you can imagine, no one is eager to take a skeptical look at the safety of these devices. Much like the tobacco industry and the connection between smoking and cancer, the strategy is "delay, delay, delay, deny, deny, deny."

They say the science is evolving. Or we need more research. Or some variation on that theme. They deny harm, while upping the volume of EMFs we all swim in. 5G, the so-called fifth generation of enhanced wireless device power, will result in all us of being exposed to some multiple of the EMFs we're already bombarded with.

And that's saying something, because manmade EMF levels are already ten billion times as high as they were in the 1960s, according to one source. Plenty of research shows all is not well, and 5,000 studies now provide evidence against the "it's harmless" theory.

Animal studies yield scary conclusions

The highly respected International Agency for Research on Cancer (IARC) classified EMFs as a class 2B "possible" carcinogen in 2011.

This classification includes wireless radiation from any transmitting source, including cell phones, baby monitors, tablets, cell towers, radar, WiFi, fitness trackers, and more. Two studies provide impressive evidence. A $25 million study by the US National Toxicology Program (NTP) observed lab rats exposed to radiation levels equivalent to a human talking 30 minutes a day on a cell phone for 36 years.

Exposed animals had higher rates of glioma brain tumors and malignant schwannoma of the heart, a very rare type of tumor. None of the unexposed animals developed these. I hardly need to point out that most people spend far more than 30 minutes a day on these devices.

This study factored heat effects, proving that nonionizing, non-heating EMFs increase cancer risk. Ironically, the whole reason NTP wanted to do this study was because senior manager John Bucher wanted to prove once and for all that cell phones do NOT cause cancer.

Instead, he added to the pile of evidence proving it does. This, for example: In 2018, the Ramazzini Institute published its sweeping lifetime study of lab rats exposed to cell tower radiation. Findings confirmed the NTP study – higher rates of heart cancer in males and brain tumors in females. Both genders had abnormally high levels of precancerous conditions.

The Ramazzini rats were exposed to radio-frequency (RF) radiation levels below the allowable maximum defined by the Federal Communications Commission (FCC). The NTP study was criticized for using higher levels. Based on the strength of these studies, scientists are encouraging IARC to rate EMFs as a "probable" carcinogen rather than a "possible" one.

Childhood leukemia

Back in the "dark ages" of 1979, researchers found a startling link between childhood leukemia and exposure to strong magnetic frequencies (MFs) created by the electric wiring in homes and by high-voltage power lines.

Note that these sources of radiation are nothing compared to wireless devices. These are just the magnetic fields that surround the physical electric wires. They quickly become weaker with distance from the source. Since then, dozens of studies have linked EMFs to cancers, including melanoma, acoustic neuroma (inner ear), breast cancer, salivary gland cancer, lymphoma, and more.

At least eight studies since 2002 show a link to brain tumors on the side of the head where the patients used their cell phones. The breast cancer link dates back to 1996. Studies revealed a higher risk for radio operators, multiple male breast cancer clusters, a three-fold risk in one study, and a seven-fold risk in another.

It takes a long while for such cancers to appear, and this works in favor of government and industry authorities that want to deny the problem. As with tobacco or pesticides or food additives, it may take decades of exposure before cancer appears.

The link is statistical. "People who were exposed to X are more likely to get cancer." And such links are easy to challenge (and sometimes the challengers are even right.) But – in a quirk that may save us from disaster – EMFs appear to cause other health problems on a much faster timetable than cancer, proving a connection that skeptics will not be able to deny. Just to give you a sneak preview: A well-executed 2017 study by Kaiser Permanente stunned researchers. Exposure for a mere 14 minutes a day during pregnancy nearly tripled risk of miscarriage.

Electro-hypersensitivity... not mental illness

Complaints of EMF sensitivity abound. Magda Havas, PhD, estimates that about 25 million people suffer extreme electro-hypersensitivity (EHS). 300 million more show signs of moderate symptoms, like headaches or insomnia. Yet doctors claim these folks are delusional, that they've gone crazy. (I can remember when they also said Lyme disease was "all in your head." Now it's known to be an infection – and an epidemic.) The Swedish government actually recognized EHS as a real medical condition since 1995. What do the Swedes know that we don't?

The most common symptoms of EHS...

- Skin problems
- Heart problems/high blood pressure
- Dizziness
- GI tract disturbances
- Sleep disorders/insomnia

- Anxiety/depression/moodiness
- Asthma/allergies
- Headaches/migraines
- Memory loss/brain fog
- Numbness
- Hearing problems/tinnitus
- Joint/muscle pain
- Fatigue
- Nausea
- Respiratory/lung disorders
- Flu symptoms
- Cramps/tremors
- Fainting/coma

Obviously, many things can cause these symptoms. But it's now known that EMFs are one of them. Interestingly, a 2015 study of 700 EHS patients found that chronic inflammation was a key factor in EHS. The participants had blood biomarkers for high histamine (allergies), low melatonin (insomnia, immune risk, and cancer), anti-myelin antibodies (muscle weakness and tingling), and oxidative stress (disease in general).

Still think it's all in their heads? There's more: the same biomarkers are found in animals exposed to EMFs. Another study found that the closer you live to a cell tower, the stronger your symptoms. The authors suggest living at least 300 meters away. That's becoming hard to do, since the number of towers has literally exploded over the past 15 years, and it'll only get worse with the rollout of 5G.

Plunging sperm counts in men

EMFs may be a powerful contraceptive, albeit one you didn't figure on. They blast your reproductive organs every moment you carry your cell phone in your pocket or use your laptop on your lap. Research shows that using a laptop on your lap, especially with WiFi turned on, reduces sperm count and motility and increases sperm DNA damage.11 Just four hours of exposure causes one-fourth of a man's sperm to become useless. No wonder so many couples find it hard to conceive a child.

Other studies confirm this finding. And an animal study showed that exposure to EMFs decimated testosterone levels. Based on a 2013 study, cell phone use may also be linked to erectile dysfunction. Men, in case you don't give two hoots about your fertility, you might want to know that your sperm quality is closely linked to your overall health. Men with high sperm counts enjoy greatly increased longevity compared to men with low counts.

Invites female reproductive havoc

EMFs also affect women's sexual functions. One study compared 180 female workers exposed to EMFs with 349 unexposed controls. The EMF group had higher rates of menstrual disorders, heavier bleeding, and reduced progesterone.

I mentioned above the study showing nearly three times the rate of miscarriage among women who were exposed to EMFs just a few minutes a day while pregnant. And ladies, while a man's sperm reserve renews itself every 74 days, the 300,000 eggs you were born with are not replenishable. Your body doesn't make new ones.

Sam Milham, MD, in his book Dirty Electricity, recounts how Dave Stetzer visited a bank where many female clerks suffered fertility problems or miscarriages. He found high levels of Dirty Electricity (DE), and remediated it with special filters. About a year later, the bank manager called, angry because too many of his workers left at the same time for maternity leave.

Choose your brain over your smartphone

Many people assume their skull protects their brain. Not so. It's not some incredible EMF-proof shell. Radiation enters your brain every time you use your devices. Ample evidence shows dire effects on your mood, memory, eyes, and ears... even at levels far below FCC guidelines.

• Martin Pall, PhD, the VGCC guy from Part One of this series, found 26 studies linking EMFs with psychiatric effects. Five of these showed EMFs were definitely the cause.

• Increased anxiety, depression, and even suicidal ideation, possibly due to stripping your brain of the neurotransmitter GABA.

• DNA neuron damage, linked to brain fog.

• Cataracts in otherwise-healthy military service members who'd been exposed to radar radiation at cell phone frequencies. 23 Glasses with metal frames make it worse, concentrating EMFs that bounce off your phone.

• An epidemic of hearing loss among teenagers in India -- on the same ear they hold their phone next to.

• A strong link to tinnitus in military personnel who work near radars... known as the "Frey" effect.

• Nervous system – exposure on the left side of the brain slows right hand reaction time, same for the right side. (The left side of the brain controls the right hand, the right side of the brain controls the left hand.)

• Damages myelin sheaths that protect your nerves.

• May be a factor in ALS (Lou Gehrig's disease) and MS (multiple sclerosis).

• Alzheimer's patients have depleted GABA and excess calcium in the brain. Both conditions are linked to EMFs. Swiss researchers found a dramatic increase in the rate of Alzheimer's in those living close to high voltage power lines.

One of the most telling factors in weight control is your blood sugar. A 2008 paper by Magda Havas showed that dirty electricity (DE) makes it harder to control blood sugar. At least five studies link radio frequency (RF) and DE to high blood glucose levels.

EMFs boost cortisol (stress hormone) levels, which are strongly correlated with waist size. Even miniscule amounts of RF radiation can trigger heart problems – high blood pressure, high heart rate, oxidative damage, calcium metabolism, and heart failure.

The Lancet, a prestigious medical journal, reported that talking on a cell phone boosts blood pressure by 5 to 10 mm. Prof. Martin Pall proposes that EMF-damaged calcium channels at the cellular level may be a central cause of heart failure.

The evidence suggests that there's no place on your body where it's safe to hold your cell phone or other device. If the phone is near your abdomen, EMFs weaken beneficial bacteria and strengthen invaders like viruses and parasites. Dr. Dietrich Klinghardt found that candida and mold cultures spew up to 600 times more biotoxins when exposed to EMFs. Apparently, these microbes feel threatened by the invisible signals we ignore, so they throw out as much poison as possible. Two other studies confirmed this. Then a shocking 2017 study showed that toxic E. coli and listeria bacteria developed resistance to antibiotics when exposed to EMFs.

Protect your little ones

Your baby absorbs far more energy per pound of body weight than you do. A one-year-old absorbs twice as much as an adult. If you want your children to outlive you, it's a very bad idea to let them have or play with a cell phone. Or tablet. Or computer. Or other high-tech gadgets.

Besides being likely causes of infertility and miscarriages, EMFs pummel unborn babies, who are developing at hyper speed. Imagine the results of DNA mistakes at this critical time. As an example, an unborn baby produces 250,000 nerve cells every minute during the entire pregnancy.

EMFs blast the blood-brain barrier, significantly increasing the risk of ADHD for children up to age seven. Some researchers ask what kind of neurological damage we're doing to kids by surrounding them with 30 iPads in a classroom... and planting 5G cell towers right on the school's roof?

Benefits of pomegranate

Forget the "an apple a day" mantra... this could be far better. On the outside, it looks somewhat like a large apple – red in color, but closer to a perfect sphere. If you've never eaten this fruit, get ready for a fun surprise -- the amazing little morsels hidden on the inside of its tough skin! They're ruby-red, translucent and shiny, so they really do look like little jewels – rubies you can eat, with a delicious sweet-tart flavor and a slight crunch.

What's more, they pack a nutritional wallop, as people knew very well in ancient times. In the Bible, these little marvels were noted for their healing properties. Some scholars suggest it might have been the forbidden fruit in the garden of Eden (the Bible merely says "fruit"; it doesn't specify what kind).

I don't know if this is what got Adam and Eve in trouble, but for you it could be a source of vibrant health. The inside of a pomegranate is a marvel to behold – a multitude of plump little red seeds separated by cream-colored membranes. Tradition states that a pomegranate contains 613 seeds. I've never counted them, so I can't confirm or deny that. The pomegranate is renowned for supporting heart health and lowering blood pressure, but today let's check out its anticancer powers.

Stops cancer in its tracks

Scientists believe certain compounds in pomegranate can stall cancer formation and progression. These compounds – punicalagin, luteolin, ellagitannins, and a variety of polyphenols – serve to obstruct many of the steps involved in cancer formation and proliferation. What's more, pomegranate doesn't offer merely one single mechanism to block cancer. Its compounds go after multiple targets.

One of the fruit's primary benefits is to turn off genes that trigger inflammation – such as NF-kappaB.1,2 This stops cancer cells from forming in the first place. A study showed that pomegranate significantly reduced tumor formation in the lungs of mice exposed to cigarette smoke over a long period of time. 3 Other studies show similar reductions in breast tumors in mice exposed to the carcinogen DMBA, found in cigarette smoke and overcooked meats.

Impairs cancer growth

Pomegranate blocks existing cancer cells from spreading in several ways:

- Interrupts the cell cycle – shuts off cancer cells' ability to divide... but does not block healthy cells' normal cell division.
- Induces cell death (apoptosis).
- Limits angiogenesis (the formation of new blood vessels that tumors grow to feed themselves).
- Prevents cancer spread – inhibits the expression of genes related to invasion, migration, and metastasis of cancer cells.

Slows prostate cancer

Pomegranate shows great promise in its ability to fight prostate cancer. One study showed that the polyphenol punicalagin blocks the growth of human prostate cancer cells, and also induces apoptosis.4 A second study confirmed the finding on apoptosis.

A different animal study looked at those with impaired immune function, and found the compounds luteolin, punicic acid, and ellagic acid significantly inhibited the growth and spread of highly invasive prostate tumors. None of the mice that consumed pomegranate experienced tumor spread, and their tumors were 25% smaller. But tumors metastasized in five of the seven mice that weren't fed pomegranate.

Human studies show its ability to slow the rise of PSA levels in men who'd been treated for prostate cancer. Prior to eating regular helpings of pomegranate, patients' PSA levels were rising, a sign of cancer progression. Post-pomegranate, their levels began to drop, indicating a significant decrease in the cancer's growth rate. A subsequent study confirmed those results. Additional studies are still needed, but based on what we know so far, pomegranate looks to be a low-cost and highly effective natural remedy.

A Godsend against numerous cancers

Studies show that pomegranate can prevent breast cancer cell growth, as well as induce cancer cell death, block inflammation, and inhibit cancer spread. One study found that pomegranate blocked the carcinogenic effects of a toxin given to the research animals, suggesting its power to prevent.

There's more: Studies confirm pomegranate's ability to fight leukemia, as well as cancers of the bladder, brain, cervix, colon/rectum, liver, lungs, ovaries, skin, and thyroid. If you opt for chemotherapy, you'll be happy to know that pomegranate can protect from chemo's nasty side effects, particularly the damage it does to the intestinal lining.15 The fruit may even enhance the cancer-killing potency of the drugs.

This fruit may be an all-natural gift from God for fighting many types of cancer, as well as for enhancing the effectiveness of other treatments. Those concerned about cancer should consume pomegranates when they're available fresh – or, when the fresh fruit is out of season, supplement with a pomegranate extract standardized to 30% punicalagin and 22% punicic acid.

If you've never purchased one of these exotic fruits, don't be flummoxed about what to do with it. You cut it in half, then in quarters, and dig out the ruby-like seeds, called arils. They're about the size of an unpopped popcorn kernel. You can eat them just as they are, like candy.

The power of combos for prostate and breast cancers

When it comes to pomegranate's influence on prostate cancer, the research results have been complicated and a bit controversial. You see, while the initial tests with pomegranate juice and extracts for prostate cancer looked very promising, further research indicates that the natural chemicals in pomegranate seem to help only certain men with prostate cancer.

What all that means: In reviewing tests of pomegranate compounds on men suffering prostate cancer, researchers from UCLA and Johns Hopkins believe that these antioxidant chemicals, when consumed all by themselves, may only be beneficial for men with prostate cancer who are over the age of 70 and who have a certain genetic makeup.

Please note, this study related to men who already have prostate cancer. It says nothing about the potential of pomegranate for preventing prostate cancer. But the secret to unlocking pomegranate's prostate benefits for a wider group of men may be to combine its nutrients with other important natural chemicals. Exciting new research out of England suggests that mixing pomegranate extract with other known cancer-fighting nutrients found in green tea, broccoli and turmeric makes pomegranate more effective in slowing down the progression of prostate cancer.

So what that says to me is that men concerned about their prostates should be eating a healthy diet containing all of these types of foods, as well as considering supplementation, to get a synergistic benefit that may be able to lower their risk of cancer.

Studies show that pomegranate can restrain breast cancer cells from multiplying and induce the cancer cells to undergo apoptosis – the programmed cell death that is designed to eliminate the body's malfunctioning cells. Studies at UCLA demonstrate that pomegranate compounds stop the action of an enzyme that can otherwise stimulate the growth of cancer cells and lead to the spread of tumors. At the same time, other research shows that the natural chemicals in this fruit can have epigenetic effects—they stimulate the genes in cancer cells that promote apoptosis, i.e. self-destruction. These pomegranate chemicals also shut down the genes that could otherwise help the cancer cells survive by repairing its DNA and making the cells multiply faster.

Overall, pomegranate is a great example of how a natural food can contain a collection of natural chemicals that offer enough benefits to keep medical researchers busy for quite a while. Perhaps more exciting, its health effects go beyond cancer. A study showed that when pomegranate compounds enter the digestive tract they help cut back on cancer-linked inflammation. In doing so, they also defend the intestinal lining from damaging conditions like ulcerative colitis and Crohn's Disease.

One key to this defense, say the researchers, is that the probiotic bacteria in the digestive tract convert pomegranate nutrients into what's called Urolithin A (UroA). And UroA, in turn, increases the accumulation of proteins that tighten up the web of cells that line the intestines and keep toxins out of the body. That helps protect against colitis and cellular damage.

A couple of cautions

Pomegranate can lower blood pressure. It may also cause dangerous side effects when combined with certain medications, such as blood thinners (e.g. warfarin) and angiotensin-converting enzyme inhibitors. Consult your doctor first if you take any of these medications. This warning applies more to concentrated pomegranate than to the raw arils. Pomegranate juice is widely available in supermarkets year-round. The juice delivers a far bigger dose, faster, than the arils.

Stress and anger - a vicious cycle

Advice from a cancer survivor: *Lose the anger.* The last panelist to tell his story about overcoming cancer was Ryan Luelf. Married for 19 years with three children, ages 7, 9, and 18, he said he was turning 39. He gave this advice to other patients who are struggling with cancer:

"Stop being angry. Stop being pissed off about what happened years ago. Remember, life flows downstream. Don't paddle against the current. Toss the oars aside, and get in the flow.

"Tune into your own infinite intelligence to find your own path, and then share it with others to help them find theirs. Drop out of your head into a deeper place within you. Get deep! D on't live out of your ego or else you'll miss the present moment. The present moment is all we have, and it's always all we have.

"Don't be lost in thoughts about the future or the past. Be

in 'the now.' Bring all your awareness about what you're doing."

In 2015 Ryan began suffering from night sweats and swollen lymph nodes in his neck. Then he came down with horrible headaches. He found out he had stage four non-Hodgkins lymphoma with metastasis from the liver to the bone marrow.

That very instant, he decided he was going to live, period. He had a wife and children who needed him. He said, "NOTHING is more powerful than deciding what your destiny is."

Ryan's doctor told him, "This cancer will kill you. You'll do chemo, but it could kill you in the first two weeks. If you don't do chemo, you'll be dead in two or three months."

This is how he replied to that doctor: "That's not going to work for me." He told the cancer patients in the audience, "Don't make an agreement with a human being's opinion. Instead, form an opinion that will serve you well, and believe it."

Ryan never thought he would die from the cancer, but he knew it was possible, and he was at peace with it. His wife, on the other hand, was stressed out. Instead of ignoring the elephant in the living room, he told his wife, "It's time to talk about the possibility that I might die and face it and deal with it."

They had long talks. He got his financial affairs in order to make sure his family was provided for. Going through this process wasn't a sign of defeat but an honorable and respectful course of action. One day his wife looked him in the eye and told him, "If you die, the kids and I will be okay." He felt relieved when his wife gave him permission to die, which gave him permission to be fully alive and in the present.

Needing $30,000 for his alternative treatment plan in a Tijuana cancer clinic, Ryan rolled up his sleeves and raised it by not being afraid to ask others for help. Based on his experience, he's developed a reasonably priced fundraising course which is for sale to cancer patients and others on the website FreelyFunded.com. When he set up a crowdfunding website, 800 people donated, enabling him to get the treatment he needed. Just for the heck of it, and with his wife's permission, he decided to do something wild. He sold their house, bought an RV, and took off on an adventure traveling the U.S. Now he's ready to settle down and buy a house in Tulsa.

Remarkable benefits of a juice fast

Using colloquial, PG-13 language, cancer coach Jill Schneider described her journey to healing from malignant cervical cancer back in the 1970s. Her doctors wanted to hustle her onto the operating table for a hysterectomy, but she refused. Instead, she experienced profound healing in a jungle in Venezuela and in the mountains of Peru.

She took herbs from a doctor of Chinese medicine and purified her blood by going on a brown rice diet for ten days. Then she added vegetables to the brown rice plus nuts, seeds, and beans. She hiked in the mountains and felt wonderful. She actually forgot that she had a cancer diagnosis.

When she ran out of money, she came back to America -- and her tests were normal. Jill advises cancer patients first to address the physical causes: dehydration, exhaustion, and malnutrition. "Fix those first before you do anything. It's a great start. Malnutrition is fixed by juicing. Everyone should do a juice fast. Fasting is holy. The kitchen is the holiest place in my house."

At retreats she does massage and promotes relaxation and sleep. She said, "We need the sugar from fruit for our brain. You have to clean out your colon. Clean it out. Get that s--t out! Usually people lose about a pound a day during a fast. If you have digestive problems, stop eating!

"Start with a three to five day fast. You're going to feel like s--t the first few days, but don't be afraid of it. Accept it. Enjoy it. Watch comedies. Try to laugh your *ss off during the first few days. Break the fast with salad, watermelon, and avocado. You're going to get your youth back and your mojo back!"

Jill is located in Delray Beach. Her website is www.circle-of-life.net. No such thing as a free lunch, right? Wrong! Keynote speaker Dr. Mary Hardy, M.D., suggested an option that, for many, might make more sense than cannabis: medicinal mushrooms. She said, "Medicinal mushrooms are as close to a free lunch as you can get: medicinal benefits without side effects."

Dr. Hardy has mentioned several mushrooms she likes, including Reishi (Ganoderma), Coriolus (Turkey Tail), Shiitake, and a mushroom extract called AHCC. It has been said that whether you have a disease or not, everybody should be on two medicinal mushrooms — reishi and cordyceps — because of their wide-ranging medical benefits for various organs and the immune system. Several reputable companies sell these mushroom extracts, including Mushroom Wisdom, Fungi Perfecti, and Mushroom Science.

Benefits of ALA

Berkson had six years of education above his medical training — a Master's and PhD in microbiology and cell biology — and was always searching for new discoveries. So he called the National Institutes of Health and spoke to the head of Internal Medicine, Dr. Fred Bartter — and asked if there was anything he knew of that could regenerate a liver.

Dr. Bartter said he was studying alpha lipoic acid because he knew it could reverse diabetic neuropathy and other complications of diabetes. But he was seeing something even more startling: when he gave it to people, it seemed to regenerate their organs. It seemed to stimulate their stem cells and start the growth of new organ tissue.

Dr. Bartter had the lipoic acid sent to Dr. Berkson, who picked it up at the Cleveland airport three hours later. The pilot handed it off to him. He raced back to the hospital and injected it into the two gravely ill patients for a period of two weeks.

By the end of those two weeks, they'd completely regenerated their livers. (And they're still alive and well, in their 80s — thirty-some years later.) Dr. Berkson was all excited. So was Dr. Bartter. But the chiefs were very upset. They said, "We told the families that these people were going to die, that there was no hope. And now they're alive and well. You know, it makes us look bad. And you did something without asking us for permission."

Berkson said, "You told me that these people were my responsibility, so I did what I thought was correct. Do you want to know what I did?" "No." They continued, "This is not an approved drug. And it's not on our formulary. And you did not follow orders like a good internal medicine doctor." "I guess I became the medical outlaw"

Dr. Berkson was chagrined. This was all very different from what he'd experienced as professor of biology. There, when he discovered something new, everyone would pat him on the back and give him awards. In medicine, if you discovered something new, you were considered some kind of outlaw.

Anyway, he was told not to do this again. But other patients came in with mushroom poisoning. There's not much you can do in this case except transplant — or take alpha lipoic acid. After achieving such remarkable results with four patients, Dr. Bartter and several other doctors flew to Cleveland and set up a national conference on organ regeneration. Young Dr. Berkson was the lead speaker.

Eventually Dr. Bartter and Dr. Berkson published a paper on 79 people with so-called terminal liver disease. Of those, 75 regenerated their livers with just intravenous lipoic acid. Doctors in the United States were almost totally uninterested. But the two authors were invited to Europe as visiting scientists at the prestigious Max Planck Institute, so they published in Europe.

When was alpha lipoic acid discovered? Sixty years ago, a team of scientists led by Dr. Lester Reed, from the University of Texas in Austin, made a startling discovery. They isolated a compound that could alter the metabolism of glucose. The term lipoic refers to 'lipid' or fat, so they named it alpha-lipoic acid (ALA).

Hundreds of articles have been published on it. At first the focus was on its role in sugar metabolism. All that changed in the 1980s — when ALA's powerful antioxidant capabilities were discovered and became the new focus of research. Researchers also became interested in alpha lipoic acid for its ability to fight various diseases and health problems:

- Protecting from infections
- Fighting inflammation
- Protecting nerve cells
- Treating cardiovascular diseases
- Fighting Cancer
- Reducing allergies
- Shielding against stomach ulcers

Alpha lipoic is a fabulous antioxidant, offering some benefits not found in other antioxidants. A leading scientist in antioxidant chemistry, Lester Packer, PhD, from the University of California-Berkeley, published a review article in the journal Free Radical Biology and Medicine in 1995 — in which he reports on the uniqueness of alpha lipoic acid.

Packer comes close to naming it the 'ideal' antioxidant because:

- ALA is readily absorbed from your diet or when taken as a supplement
- It has the uncanny ability to regenerate 'used-up' vitamin C, extending C's value way beyond normal.
- It can potentially regenerate other antioxidants.
- It increases your levels of glutathione, your primary cellular antioxidant. (More on this in a moment.)
- ALA can help replenish your body's vitamin E

Are you what you eat?

"You are what you eat" has become a common adage. And it's true. The food you eat impacts your health and wellbeing directly. Vegetables and fruits supply you with numerous vitamins, minerals and antioxidants, as well as fiber. Natural carbs like those produced by green plants through photosynthesis provide you with sugars your cells burn for energy.

Your mitochondria function as the powerhouses of your cells, producing the energy required for life. The mitochondrion is actually a package of enzymes responsible for the slow and orderly burning of food with oxygen. Cells with high energy requirements — like your heart and liver cells — have abundant mitochondria. One microscopic liver cell can contain more than 2,000 mitochondrial powerhouses.

All the food you eat is eventually converted to sugar and used as fuel for the mitochondrion. It's in this context that ALA does one of its most important jobs. Without alpha lipoic acid, the prepared glucose cannot enter the mitochondrion. So, no ALA — no energy produced — and no life. You aren't what you eat, because it never gets utilized.

Therefore, ALA is necessary to keep you alive. Interestingly, ALA's structure allows it to be both water-soluble and fat-soluble — making it a superb detoxifying antioxidant. One of ALA's major roles is to transfer sugar into your powerhouse mitochondrion. It's impossible to move that fuel across the membrane without ALA.

ALA and the aging process

A major cause of aging is free radical damage. Free radical molecules contain uneven numbers of electrons, making them highly unstable. They're forever trying to stabilize themselves by stealing electrons from stable molecules. Stable molecules coming in contact with free radicals are always in danger of losing an electron to this unstable electron thief, causing a chain reaction that destroys the delicate structure of the cell.

Fortunately you can control and counter this destructive process, at least in part. You can effectively delay aging by following Dr. Berkson's five rules of healthy living, outlined in The Alpha Lipoic Acid Breakthrough: The Superb Antioxidant:

- Eat a healthy, largely vegetable diet, enhanced with

nutritional supplements. Don't overeat.

- Get on a regular exercise program.
- Get 7-8 hours sleep per night.
- Limit your exposure to environmental toxins – alcohol, cigarette smoke, smog, industrial chemicals, radiation, prescription drugs, etc.
- Relieve your stress

Supplementing with antioxidants can help protect you from free radical bombardment. What makes ALA such a potent antioxidant? ALA works double duty. It seeks and heals free radical damage in every setting – whether in brain fluids, your blood, stored fat, your heart, pancreas, kidneys, bone, cartilage, liver... or any other cell in any organ of your body, for that matter.

It is both a hydrophilic and lipophilic molecule. In simple terms, that means it's water-soluble and fat-soluble – explaining why it does double duty. These remarkable characteristics allow it to pass through the blood-brain barrier – so it increases brain energy.

ALA has a fabulous ability... It can salvage and recycle other antioxidants like vitamin C, vitamin E and glutathione. Whenever one of these antioxidants is used up, ALA can renew its effectiveness – letting those antioxidants do double duty too. Biochemists call this antioxidant recycling.

Also, ALA protects collagen in your skin, preventing wrinkling and the appearance of aging in your body. Further, it guards your DNA and RNA from damage, neutralizing potentially dangerous chemicals that trigger gene expression leading to cancer.

Last but not least, ALA encourages your body to produce glutathione – an indispensable and powerful antioxidant within your cells. Glutathione protects your body from free radical damage. It defends against free radical waste products – as well as toxins produced by alcohol consumption, cigarette smoking, cancer chemotherapy, and exposure to damaging radiation.

Dr. David Williams, a well known authority on alternative medicine regarded glutathione as a critical anti-aging nutrient, but our levels go down as we age. In his opinion, the higher your glutathione levels, the longer you're likely to live. Many patients with diseases have low glutathione levels.

Dr. Keith Scott-Mumby regards glutathione as critical to liver health, and good liver health is critical to overall good health. The problem is, you can't supplement directly with glutathione because it's broken down in the stomach. Dr. Williams says the same thing. Since it's useless to take straight glutathione supplements, you need to supplement with the building blocks of glutathione. Then your body will have what it needs to manufacture glutathione for itself. One of those key building blocks is alpha lipoic acid.

As Dr. Berkson found in his research, your liver can regenerate itself if you give it the tools, including alpha lipoic acid. But you need other nutrients, too. Glutathione's ability to guard against free radical damage extends not only to your liver but also to your blood vessels, nervous system, immune system, lungs and kidneys.

ALA and radiation

Nuclear radiation is a huge promoter of free radicals with high potential to kill you. In animal experiments, ALA was shown to protect the bone marrow of mice from radiation injuries. One of the worst nuclear accidents in history occurred in Chernobyl, Russia in 1986. It exposed local residents to constant radiation. Soil was contaminated more than 1,000 miles away. The Russian government administered ALA by itself and also with vitamin E — and reported that abnormal liver and kidney functions became normal again with ALA.

Alpha lipoic acid as a chelating agent

The fact that ALA can reverse radiation damage suggests it might also function as a chelation agent for heavy metals such as lead and mercury. Certain substances can grasp and bind metals, neutralize them, and carry them out of your system. Excessive heavy metals can cause oxidative stress (basically, free radical damage), and promote unhealthy changes, kill healthy cells, or lead to disease. Some heavy metals, like mercury and arsenic, can cause serious organ damage.

Alpha lipoic acid chelates mercury, arsenic, copper, excess iron, cadmium, excess calcium, zinc and lead. Dr. Lester Packer continues to do exciting research on antioxidant biochemistry. But the research so far suggests that ALA is a great therapeutic agent for heavy metal poisoning. Can ALA treat or prevent cancer?

Traditional medicine's view of cancer treatment continues to consist of surgery, chemotherapy, and radiation... despite the incredible discoveries of natural cures in the past twenty years. Dr. Berkson notes that sensible cell biologists know everyone forms cancer cells during their lifetime, but only 30% are diagnosed with clinical cancer — suggesting that you're born with the capacity to destroy cancer cells using your immune system... and that disease occurs when something disrupts your normal immune response. Though cancer usually develops over a long time period, the disease begins with damage to either genes or mitochondria in a cell — along with a weakened immune system that allows these abnormal cells to proliferate.

Treating cancer

The first — and best — line of defense against cancer is a good offense... through a sound, high-antioxidant, mostly raw diet full of nourishing enzymes. Dr. Berkson believes that despite the grim prospects painted for cancer, there's mounting scientific evidence that various nutrients can stop and possibly reverse cancer. But be aware, it's a very rare day when a doctor will give you a nutritional plan to prevent cancer. That starts and ends with you!

Can ALA discourage cancer?

Alpha lipoic acid is a potent antioxidant that's incredibly effective at stopping free radicals and dangerous toxins from taking over. It's been reported to neutralize the toxic effects of radiation therapy in animal studies, and shown to alleviate harmful effects of chemo in cancer patients.

Scientists speculate that ALA might actually discourage cancer development, or may reverse or hold off the malignant syndrome. In very simple terms, it does that by stopping the damaging messages that flow from messenger molecules outside of cells to the nucleus inside cells. It appears ALA can do this both indirectly by quenching free radicals, and directly by stabilizing these messengers.

This is exciting because — if true — it means ALA can potentially stop cells that are genetically programmed to become cancerous, causing them to remain non-cancerous.

Vitamins needed for ALA to perform well

As often happens, one nutrient (or hormone, or whatever) does not operate solo. ALA works better when combined with various vitamins. Vitamin A - Is shown to reduce the risk of many cancers by supporting immune function. Sometimes used as a complementary treatment with conventional cancer therapy. Upholds the integrity of your skin, mucous membranes, and other barriers to invading alien cells.

Vitamin C - improves the strength of your blood. Can destroy cancer cells, neutralize toxins that can influence cancer, and strengthen your immune system. And remember — ALA can recycle and reuse used-up vitamin C. With ALA, vitamin C works over and over.

Vitamin E - Works in fatty environments. Helps prevent normal cells from becoming cancerous. ALA recycles vitamin C, which in turn recycles used-up vitamin E. So both vitamin C and E are optimized in the presence of ALA. Be aware that too much vitamin E can be harmful, according to some experts.

Glutathione - The most important intra-cellular antioxidant. Mops up toxins and free radicals. Forms systems that defend against cancer-causing free radicals. ALA has been shown to increase production of and recycle glutathione.

Selenium - Found through eating green leafy plants. Scientists believe selenium fights cancer directly as a powerful antioxidant, and indirectly by increasing glutathione activity. You need small amounts to stay healthy. But caution — selenium is toxic in large amounts.

Taking alpha lipoic acid

Because it's such a potent antioxidant, it seems logical to consider taking ALA along with other supplements you take. ALA is readily available at health food and supplement stores. The ideal dose of ALA has not been established. Dr. Berkson stresses that the proper dose varies from one person to another, and you should develop your ALA plan with the help of a well-informed doctor who is truly committed to disease prevention. Reminder: ALA will do the most for you in the context of eating at least six servings of fresh fruits and veggies per day. Which form should you take? R-ALA is more potent than the commonly sold synthetic ALA which usually contains both the R and S forms. The S form is a mirror image of the R form and not easily utilized by the body.

The bottom line

Alpha lipoic acid is an exciting addition to the list of nutrients, herbs and hormones that can treat disease in a safer, more natural way than conventional drugs — and help you to become healthier. But, as with any medicine, ALA is not a magic bullet that can cure disease in the face of poor diet, lack of exercise and other lifestyle choices. Your body — like everyone's — is complicated, involving countless biochemical reactions occurring at every moment. Give ALA its due, but use it as one part of an overall strategy for maximum health. That is when ALA can really shine.

PSA and other testing tools

A screening tool that lacks precision. Totally unnecessary treatment. Poor prognostic tools. Men certainly draw the short straw when it comes to prostate cancer. With 174,650 American men expected to receive a prostate cancer diagnosis in 2019, urgently needed are better methods of early detection, more reliable ways to predict an individual's likely outcome, and improved treatments. Prostate cancer is not considered confirmed until the man has a biopsy, a procedure in which small samples of tissue are cut out and examined in a lab.

By all accounts it's a nasty, uncomfortable procedure that can cause bleeding and pain in the days following. It also risks hospitalization due to infection. In addition to these downsides, three out of ten biopsies result in a false negative. "False negative" means the test shows you're cancer-free – when in fact you're not.

Appalling, but even after submitting to this invasive,

damaging procedure the diagnosis may be wrong. In the standard transrectal ultrasonography-guided biopsy of the prostate, the doctor takes ten to twelve random samples (cores) from the organ. But this approach under-detects clinically significant cancers that need treatment, and over-detects low grade cancers that don't need to be treated.

So researchers are exploring a new method to see whether a biopsy is required at all, and if so, to take cores from suspicious tissue only. It's called multiparametric magnetic resonance imaging (MRI) -- cutting edge technology that can produce a detailed image of the prostate. In a major study published in the New England Journal of Medicine last year, 500 men at 25 centers in 11 countries were randomized to receive either an MRI-targeted biopsy or a standard biopsy.

The former detected 46 percent more clinically significant, and 59 percent less clinically insignificant cancers than the latter, and it did so with far fewer biopsy cores, meaning less potential for harm. 71 of 252 men (28%) had MRI results that suggested there was no prostate cancer, so those patients didn't undergo a biopsy. Veeru Kasivisvanathan, the first author of the large research team, said, "This is the first trial in which men who have a negative MRI have had a chance to avoid biopsy altogether."

High hopes for the new approach

Another member of the team was consultant urologist Mark Emberton, Professor of Interventional Oncology at University College London. He has spent ten years investigating the new technology and is very enthusiastic about it: "MRI for all men prior to biopsy of the prostate is the most important development in the management of men with early prostate cancer that we have had in the last 100 years."

Declan Murphy, director of genitourinary oncology at the Peter MacCallum Cancer Center in Melbourne, Australia, who was not involved with the study, was also upbeat about the findings. In his view, "This is an incredibly important, practice-changing study, and we need to fast-forward MRI to the diagnostic pathway prior to biopsy."

The UK's National Institute for Health and Care Excellence (NICE) was so impressed by the research, last December they recommended all men at risk of prostate cancer receive an MRI scan ahead of a biopsy. This will now be introduced across Britain's National Health Service.

Make an informed decision

Prostate cancer is usually diagnosed later in life, and in most cases progresses so slowly that, as doctors admit, more men die with prostate cancer than from it. But in a minority of cases – about one out of ten, from what I can learn -- prostate cancer can be aggressive and life-threatening.

Technology hasn't advanced enough to make accurate predictions about which tumors will grow quickly and spread beyond the prostate, and which ones will develop slowly and remain confined. This makes it difficult for the patient to know whether or not to opt for the conventional treatments – surgery, radiation and chemotherapy.

A study published in the New England Journal of Medicine in 2016 found those whose cancer was confined to the prostate and who were categorized as low or medium risk did not reap any benefit from surgery or radiotherapy over the following ten years compared to patients who refused these treatments and opted for "watchful waiting." Men in both groups had equal chance of survival. And obviously, the untreated men avoided the horrible side effects of the conventional treatments.

New way to predict if prostate cancer is dangerous

To help both clinicians and patients decide whether to closely monitor tumors or to opt for treatment, an evidence-base web tool called PREDICT Prostate was created by researchers at

Cambridge University, England. Taking all diagnostic tests, age, and medical history into account, the tool provides an estimate for ten- to 15-year survival. It also takes the likelihood of treatment success and the risk of side effects into account, and provides a survival estimate based on each of the chosen options.

The tool was developed using a high-quality database of 10,000 UK men, and validated in 2,500 cancer patients in Singapore. The approach was 90% accurate at predicting the chances of dying. According to Vincent Gnanapragasam, a consultant urologist at the University of Cambridge, "When men are diagnosed with prostate cancer and are deciding what to do they are often given wishy-washy advice which hugely depends on who they have spoken to. Our work puts a number on it to help guide those decisions. "I would say 30 percent or more of men diagnosed with prostate cancer may not benefit from treatment, based on our models. When men see their absolute risk of dying is quite low, they find it easier to decide to just monitor their cancer rather than choosing treatment." Commenting on PREDICT Prostate, Dr. Iain Frame of Prostate Cancer UK said, "Too many men undergo radical treatments for prostate cancer -- and in some cases endure life-changing side effects -- for a cancer that may never cause them harm. A tool like this has tremendous potential." The tool is available at https://prostate.predict.nhs.uk

A liquid biopsy

Another option now available is a simple, non-invasive urine test for men over 50 who have a PSA reading between 2–10 ng/ml. It's called ExoDx Prostate(IntelliScore) or EPI. The test measures three important genomic RNA bio-markers that are only expressed in high-grade prostate cancer. It provides a score which corresponds to the Gleason Score, another and more common test for gauging the seriousness of a prostate cancer. EPI grades the aggressiveness of cancer in biopsied tissue, and helps both the doctor and patient decide whether a biopsy is needed. It's been clinically validated in over a thousand patients in two large trials involving leading experts. The authors of the most recent study, published in December 2018, wrote that EPI "improves identification of patients with higher grade disease and would reduce the total number of unnecessary biopsies."

Reducing side effects

One of the most common prostate cancer treatments involves directing high-energy X-ray beams at the prostate from outside the body. In a series of treatments it kills cancer cells or slows their growth, but it's hard to prevent damage to the prostate's healthy tissues. The result is unpleasant side effects -- and the potential to grow secondary tumors in the bladder or bowel. But a new procedure greatly reduces the risks. It's a firm but pliable hydrogel made from a type of flexible plastic called polyethylene glycol. The product is named Space OAR (space for organs at risk).

It's injected as a liquid into the perineum - the gap between the anus and scrotum - until it reaches the small space between the prostate and the rectum. Here it spreads over a distance of about an inch, and quickly solidifies into a soft gel to magnify the width tenfold to four-tenths of an inch. This creates a protective barrier between the prostate and the rectum. The procedure takes place about a month before radiotherapy is scheduled. After six months the gel breaks down into tiny molecules and passes out of the body. Clinical trials have shown it to be safe and effective, lowering the radiation dose to the rectum by nearly three-quarters (73.5 percent), and thereby reducing rectal and urinary complications. After 3 years, retained sexual function was 78 percent more likely to occur in Space OAR patients compared to controls.

In the control group, a clinically significant decline of these three quality of life factors (bowel, urinary, sexual) was eight times higher than among the Space OAR group. The procedure was cleared by the FDA several years ago and is currently being used in many leading cancer centers throughout the United States. Victor Tomlinson, MD, radiation oncologist at AnMed Health Medical Center in Anderson, South Carolina said the new procedure has "really changed the game in prostate cancer care. We've had great success with this product and it's worked every time we've used it." Douglas Brown, MD, radiation oncologist at Cowell Family Cancer Center in Traverse City, Michigan, was equally positive, saying "the results are phenomenal. This is a real game-changer for patients. It essentially eliminates one of the most feared toxicities of radiation, and that's injury to the rectum."

Targeted treatment

X-rays targeted at the prostate from outside the body damage healthy tissue because they release energy both before and after they hit their target. Proton beams however, release the bulk of their energy only when they hit the prostate gland. The protons themselves are subatomic, positively-charged particles. Five trillion of them are fired every second after being 'accelerated' to two-thirds the speed of light. A small dose is delivered along the way to the prostate but virtually none beyond it. This allows more radiation to be delivered with little damage to normal tissues. It has even more advantages. It can be delivered with laser-like precision. Intensity of radiation can be varied at any point within the tumor, and involves little or no recovery time or impact on energy levels. Patients are able to work, exercise and remain sexually active both during and after treatment.

In spite of all these benefits, researchers from Harvard in a recently published review found clinical trials to date do not point to any clear advantages for proton beam therapy over conventional photon-based radiotherapy. However, as they also pointed out, this is fast moving technology and we need to await the results of trials currently in progress before we can make a final judgment. Yet many doctors who carry out the procedure are already convinced it's a step forward over conventional radiotherapy. One of these is radiation oncologist Edward Soffen, MD from Princeton Radiation Oncology, New Jersey. He calls proton therapy "one of the most advanced, sophisticated ways of treating patients with radiation. The patients who go through this form of treatment have significantly fewer side effects and they also demonstrate fewer long term issues." There are currently only 26 operational treatment centers in the US. They can be found at https://www.proton-therapy.org/map

Spoiler alert: I did not use any of the treatments in this chapter. This information was just provided as an update for information's sake If you want to supplement your treatment. Personally I needed no X-ray beam or proton therapy treatment myself.

Eating habits to prevent metastasis

What you eat and drink also affects your metastatic risk. According to biomedical engineers at Duke University, anyone with cancer should avoid foods that contain high-fructose corn syrup. There's plenty of research to back this up -- that anyone who wants to be healthy should avoid food and drinks containing corn syrup. According to the Duke studies, when cancer cells start to roam, they may seek out the liver to feast on, because fructose accumulates in that organ if your diet has been rich in high-fructose corn syrup.

The Duke study focused on cancer cells from tumors in the colon. The researchers found that although these wandering cancer cells are still genetically identical to what they were in the digestive tract, when they sense fructose in the liver, they undergo epigenetic effects – genes are activated that allow the cancer cells to gorge on the liver's supply of fructose. "Genetically speaking, colon cancer is colon cancer no matter where it goes," says researcher Xiling Shen, "but that doesn't mean that it can't respond to a new environment (like the liver). We had a hunch that such a response might not be genetic, but metabolic in nature."

Dr. Shen notes that certain metabolic genes became more active in liver metastases than they were in the original primary tumor. It seems that when the liver has been stocking up on fructose, the rich pickings stimulate the genes in the cancer cells that help them use fructose to fuel their functions. So if you've been eating the typical American diet, full of soft drinks and other sweet treats flavored with high fructose corn syrup, you are filling your body with cancer's favorite food. "When cancer cells get to the liver, they're like a kid in a candy store," warns Dr. Shen. "They use this ample new energy supply to create building blocks for growing more cancer cells."

Control stress to control cancer

While folks who study cancer have long suspected that stress can increase your risk for the spread of cancer, it's only within the last year or so that researchers have started to untangle some of the specific factors that lead from stress to metastasis. In lab tests on breast cancer conducted at the University of Basel in Switzerland, researchers discovered that the stress hormones cortisol and corticosterone interact with receptors on cancer cells that help the cells colonize other organs. The hormones also help the cells survive and proliferate in various organs around the body.

At the same time, researchers at the University of Illinois have found that epinephrine, another stress hormone, initiates a whole series of biochemical reactions that spurs on the growth of breast cancer and encourages its metastatic spread. These researchers conclude that controlling stress is a key way to control the spread of cancer. The Basel researchers suggest exercising along with relaxation techniques like meditation to limit stress. And findings by the scientists in Illinois indicate that vitamin C may help. Their lab tests found evidence that vitamin

C may be able to shrink metastatic tumors.

Don't wait to adopt these healthy habits

When researchers perform more studies on how to protect against metastases, they'll probably also find that eating a diet filled with fruits and vegetables can up the body's defenses against metastases. So far, only a few studies have found that this kind of diet reduces your risk of aggressive cancer. The evidence is not quite definitive.6 But I wouldn't wait to adopt a diet rich in fresh produce. And for sure it's a good idea to sleep in a dark bedroom, take some vitamin C, and control stress through exercise and meditation. Those habits all have multiple health benefits along with their anti-cancer characteristics. I also recommend regular milk thistle supplementation. It's healthy for many liver related reasons besides its effect on cancer.

Frankincense holy cure

There are traditional health remedies that have been around since the Bronze Age. That's the case for frankincense, which has been traded on the Arabian Peninsula for more than 6,000 years. The very word frankincense means "high quality incense." Its fragrance is a blend of piney, lemony scents melded with a sweet, woody aroma that fills traditional ritual churches on holy days like Easter and Christmas. Church-going folks also know it as one of the three gifts of the Magi to the infant Jesus.

Frankincense is a product of scraggly trees of the genus Boswellia. They grow mostly in India and Africa. When the bark is slashed from the tree, resin bleeds out and hardens into little rock-like nuggets. It's these hardened streaks of resin, called tears, which are harvested and sold. Within the tears of resin are active components called boswellic acids, which show promise against brain, prostate, bladder, cervical, and colon cancers, as well as multiple myeloma (bone marrow cancer).

The ability to fight inflammation is the main mechanism

behind the healing properties of boswellic acid. This has important implications for cancer treatment, as a large number of studies have linked inflammation to cancer. Here's just a glimpse of the many ways boswellic acid helps curb inflammation:

• It inhibits 5-lipooxygenase (5-LOX) – an inflammatory enzyme -- and may also target free radicals and cytokines that play a role in inflammation.

• In animal experiments, a boswellic acid called AKBA stands above the rest because it slashed precancerous polyps by 49% in the small intestine and by 60% in the colon. Better yet, it kept them from turning malignant. AKBA seems to stop cancer cell proliferation in several ways, most notably by inducing apoptosis – programmed cell death – by switching on the aptly named "death receptor" on cancer cell surfaces. This activates the "suicide" pathways inside cancer cells and blocks the signals cancer cells use to replicate.

• Boswellic acids help decrease brain swelling from glioblastoma, a deadly brain cancer. This means a patient may require fewer anti-inflammatory drugs. The frankincense extract can reduce or replace steroid use in brain tumors, which is important because steroids interfere with the natural death of the cancer cells. Boswellia also kills glioblastoma cells outright.

• Boswellia halts the damage caused by the 5-LOX immune system molecule, which goes rogue in certain types of cancer. In prostate tissue, 5-LOX contributes to inflammation and prostate swelling as well as cancer.

• Boswellic acids also shut down the master inflammation regulatory complex NF-kappaB in tumor cells, bringing about early tumor death and regression.

• Finally, some studies suggest that boswellia may reduce inflammation or swelling due to radiation therapy, but more studies are needed to confirm this.

To underscore the point: Reducing inflammation is one of the most important preventive strategies against cancer. But boswellic acids don't stop there. Boswellia is also known to suppress a tumor growth factor called VEGF (vascular endothelial growth factor) that cancers need to grow new blood vessels.

In addition, it may suppress tumor growth in pancreatic and colorectal cancers, and in some cases may outright prevent tumor growth (prostate and glioma). In lab-cultured pancreatic cancer cells, boswellic acid has been shown to suppress viability and induce cell death.

And in bladder cancer, boswellia has been shown to selectively kill cancer cells and leave the healthy ones alone. The compounds are able to discern the difference between healthy and cancerous tissue, so they quell tumor cells but spare normal ones.

One of the most promising natural anticancer agents

Overall, therapeutic success rates for cancer can improve dramatically with the use of boswellic acids. In fact, they currently are considered "one of the most promising anticancer agents" according to an article published in the Journal of Medical Sciences. They target multiple molecular and cellular pathways in cancer with few adverse side effects. Boswellia supplements are readily available on the Web and sometimes in retail health stores. Combining boswellia with a milk thistle derivative called silymarin is even better. The combination of the two herbs is much more potent than either one alone.

Health benefits of flaxseed

Did you know the Emperor Charlemagne, ruler of a large part of Europe in the 8th century, was so keen on flaxseed benefits that he passed laws to promote the food? Every citizen loyal to the king was expected to eat flaxseed for health. Now, twelve centuries later, we have the research to back up what Charlemagne suspected.

Flaxseed is already a popular health food. You can find it everywhere and in wide a range of products, from frozen waffles to oatmeal. Flaxseed is used to feed chickens that lay eggs said to have higher levels of omega-3 fatty acids. And well over 300 new flax-based products came out in the market over the past several years.

A tiny seed with a power-punch of health benefits

You'll find two types of flax seeds in most health food stores: brown and yellow/golden. When put through an expeller press (also known as oil pressing), they create a vegetable oil.

Both can be consumed, though brown flax oil is most commonly used in paints and for cattle feed. We know flaxseeds (also called linseeds) have high levels of both fiber and lignans, along with various micronutrients and omega-3 fatty acids. They're also high in manganese and vitamin B1.

Lignans play an important role in flaxseed's health benefits. They're a group of highly-concentrated phytochemicals found in plants. They're also part of a major class of phytoestrogens, which are basically chemicals similar to human estrogen that can act as antioxidants when consumed. Along with that, lignans have beneficial hormone-like effects on the body. Flaxseeds have a higher level of lignans than most other foods, although lignans can also be found in some cereal grains, fruits (especially strawberries and apricots), and vegetables (particularly the cruciferous ones like broccoli and cabbage).

A diet rich in flaxseed appears to lower cholesterol — especially so for women — along with helping to lower high blood pressure. The little seeds also help stabilize blood sugar levels and thereby help prevent or treat diabetes. Thanks to their dietary fiber content, they can be used to help with constipation. Flaxseed appears to be effective in reducing menopausal symptoms as well.

Flaxseed helps with cancer

Studies suggest that consuming flax seeds may benefit people with certain types of cancer, especially breast and prostate cancers. A Duke University study suggested eating flaxseed might inhibit the growth of prostate tumors. And the lignans in flaxseed are believed to cause the body to produce less active forms of estrogen, which lowers breast cancer risk. Evidence also suggests that consuming ground flaxseed on a regular basis decreases cell growth in breast tissue. Plus, animal studies have shown that both flaxseed oil and lignans can reduce breast tumor growth and the spread of cancer cells, including estrogen receptor positive (ER+) cells.

Yet, in total contrast, because flaxseed has been shown to affect intracellular signals in the body, some researchers believe it could help promote breast and prostate cancer growth. For this reason, they urge patients with ER+ breast cancer to use flaxseed with caution. Lignans are at the center of the controversy because of their potential estrogenic effects in the body. It's the same hormone-related cloud that hangs over soy products.

This controversy over the phytoestrogens in soy and flaxseed is one of the most vexing in alternative health. Those who favor the use of phytoestrogens in treating breast and prostate cancer say the phytoestrogens occupy the estrogen receptors on cancer cells without doing any harm. They elbow out human estrogen and prevent it from worsening these types of cancer. The Budwig Protocol is one of the most acclaimed and popular alternative cancer treatments. It features flaxseed oil mixed with cottage cheese. While flaxseed oil lacks the fiber, it enables you to take in a much larger dose of the lignans and omega-3s than you are ever likely to get from consuming the ground seed.

Thousands of people report controlling and even curing their cancer thanks to the Budwig Protocol. There may be some controversy where the estrogen-sensitive cancers are concerned, but for other types of cancer — and as a preventive measure — flaxseed seems to be effective. And lignans also have antiangiogenic properties, meaning they can keep tumors from forming new blood vessels. Also on the cancer-fighting front, the omega-3 fatty acids in flaxseed are believed to keep malignant cells from hanging on to other body cells.

What's better: Ground or whole flaxseed?

Most nutrition experts recommend ground flaxseed over whole. Ground flaxseed is easier for your body to digest, while whole flaxseeds can pass through your entire system and remain intact — meaning you won't get the health benefits. If you're looking for a fiber boost, always choose ground flaxseed over flaxseed oil. The fiber is found in the seed coat, which is why you're better off eating the seed itself.

A single tablespoon of ground flaxseed has roughly two grams of dietary fiber and two grams of polyunsaturated fatty acids (that includes omega 3s). A tablespoon of flax registers at only 37 calories. For the most part, flaxseed is safe to consume. There could be some complications with toxicity if you eat a massive amount, but that's true for just about any food. Note that flaxseed can act as a laxative and give you diarrhea.

You can buy both whole and ground flaxseed in bulk at most grocery stores and health food stores. If you prefer to grind your own flaxseed, a coffee grinder does the trick. Just be sure to store all ground flaxseed in an airtight container and it will last up to several months. I recommend refrigerating the seeds as well. Some easy ways to add flaxseed to your diet include:

- A tablespoon of ground flaxseed in your breakfast cereal (hot or cold)
- A tablespoon mixed into a serving of yogurt
- A tablespoon mixed into the mayonnaise or mustard on any sandwich
- Various amounts baked into breads, cookies, and muffins

Don't eat more than two or three tablespoons of ground flaxseed per day, or you might spend a lot of time in the bathroom.

Blackened meat or not

Marinate your meat before you cook it. When you marinate meat, fish or chicken for 30 minutes or more, fewer carcinogenic HCAs form when you put them on the grill. While no one is sure why this is protective, one theory is that the sugar and fat that sticks to the meat from the marinade absorbs the heat and is seared instead of the proteins in the meat. Cook your meat with spices, herbs, black or green tea, chili peppers and other botanic ingredients. The spices and other plant substances contain natural compounds called phenols -- antioxidants that can chemically react with the carcinogens that form and change them into less harmful substances. And research shows that phenols can lower the risk of diabetes, obesity and inflammation.

Don't put processed meat on the grill. Processed foods like hot dogs have been strongly linked to cancer, and researchers believe we eat too many of them. And if you thought consumption of these processed meats has gone down, think again. Americans are still eating as many hot dogs as they did a couple of decades ago. Plus, processed meat has been classified as "carcinogenic to humans" by the International Agency for Research on Cancer. It poses a danger no matter what method you use to cook it. Limit the time food is on the grill. By cooking things faster, you limit the HCAs that form. Some experts recommend baking your meat a little in the oven first before throwing it on the grill. Cutting your meat into smaller chunks can also help it cook more quickly and form fewer HCAs. Some experts advise cooking food in aluminum foil to protect the food from smoke and help it cook faster. However, research does show that cooking items in foil can leach aluminum into your food at unhealthy levels.

Grill more fruits and vegetables. Vegetarian foods don't form harmful carcinogenic chemicals the way meats do when they're grilled. Cook at lower temperatures. If you have a gas grill, don't turn the heat way up. If you're cooking over a wood fire, choose a hardwood like maple or hardwood instead of a soft wood like pine. The hardwoods don't burn as hot. Charcoal also burns at a lower temperature than softwoods. Keep a clean grill. That char that builds up on the grill? When it gets on the next burger or steak that's being cooked, it adds carcinogens to your food. So give the grill a good scrub between cooking sessions.

Don't breathe in the barbecue smoke. When you inhale the smoke coming off the grill, you may get a carcinogenic lung-full of HCAs. To cut down on your exposure, you should also wash your clothes after a barbecue. Taking a shower doesn't hurt either. Keep the fat out of the fire. Since dripping fat creates carcinogens when it falls into the fire and burns, try to cook leaner cuts of meat that don't yield as much fat. And don't poke your utensils into the cooking meats – that releases fatty juices that burn.

All charred meat is pro-cancer. AVOID them completely.

Excitotoxins and glutamate bombs

The human brain contains a chemical messenger that needs to be handled with as much care as a dangerous explosive. This molecule plays a key role in vital brain functions like learning and memory, but it has an ugly alter ego. It can also inflict massive damage if large amounts accidentally spill into your brain tissue. When a stroke, head injury, brain disease, or other injury or illness releases a flood of this substance – called glutamate – the result is damage to neurons left and right. It doesn't kill the neurons outright. Instead, it excites them to death.

Glutamate is normally kept in check by a system of dams that release it in a tiny trickle, only as needed. A stroke, head injury, or brain cancer causes those dams to burst, and glutamate floods the brain. The damage spreads outward. When it comes to glutamate, the old adage holds true that "the dose makes the poison." A small amount is good, a lot is not. Some doctors have noted that every neurological disease is mostly driven by glutamate.

GABA helps control glutamate

You can't discuss glutamate without mentioning GABA, the primary inhibitory neurotransmitter. GABA puts the brakes on glutamate's activity. But it's a bit complicated, because glutamate is actually a precursor to GABA. And the whole business also works in reverse: GABA can turn itself back into glutamate if needed. I can attest that supplementing with GABA can be tricky. For me, it's a powerful stimulant.

An excess of glutamate and the resulting excitotoxicity are triggered by: (1) too much glutamate accumulation, and (2) glutamate receptors becoming hypersensitive and over-stimulated. In reality, multiple things can go wrong, leading to glutamate excess. A flash flood of glutamate can trigger many different brain disorders, as well as things like migraines, anxiety, restlessness, inability to concentrate, insomnia (brain racing in the middle of the night), fatigue, and pain sensitivity.

How to "mop up" glutamate naturally

So is there a way to "mop up" these excess messengers naturally? The science is still evolving, but there are steps you can take today, and they're important if you're dealing with any brain conditions, including brain cancer.

1. Eliminate gluten and casein from your diet.

2. Avoid foods containing MSG (monosodium glutamate, aka "pure glutamate"). This ingredient is famously said to be common in salty and Chinese foods, but in reality it's in thousands of processed foods, and may be on the label under many different names. Whatever it's called, MSG triggers the cluster of symptoms dubbed Chinese restaurant syndrome. This pervasive food additive has a long list of reported side effects, so it's best to avoid it. For what it's worth (not much, in my view), the scientific community claims MSG is safe.

3. Reduce stress. It triggers glutamate activity.

4. Take vitamin B6. A deficiency triggers glutamate buildup and reduces GABA.

5. Reduce caffeine intake. It increases glutamate production at the expense of GABA.

6. Eat more ginger. It protects your brain from MSG-induced excitotoxicity.

7. Take vitamin C. It protects the receptors that control glutamate release.

8. Take CoQ10. It protects vulnerable brain cells from free radical damage.

9. Check out PQQ (Pyrroloquinoline Quinone) – a little-known supplement that protects the brain from glutamate toxicity.

10. Exercise. It helps optimize glutamate-to-GABA balance.

11. Eat foods rich in taurine. Taurine mimics GABA in the brain. Shellfish, poultry's dark meat, and nori (the seaweed used to wrap sushi) are rich in taurine.

Benefits of raw foods

The new mania for raw foods traces its roots back to the late 1800s when a doctor named Maximilian Bircher-Benner discovered he could cure his jaundice by eating raw apples. Since then, hundreds of experiments have been launched to test the effects of raw food on human health. These last few years, the raw food diet has become a movement (or a fad, depending on your point of view). Enthusiasts believe it will cure or prevent practically every chronic disease. I don't go that far, but it does have some real benefits. Even if you don't go for it whole-hog, here are some reasons why you should make at least a half-way move toward a whole-food diet.

A true raw food diet means you eat food that hasn't been changed in any way from its natural form. That means you stay away from anything that's cooked, processed, microwaved, irradiated, or genetically modified by high-tech gene-splicing, as well as anything grown with pesticides or herbicides. The result is a diet that consists mostly of organic, fresh fruits, berries, nuts, seeds, herbs, and vegetables. Several variations to the diet exist, but typical raw-food enthusiasts allocate 75% to 80% of their daily diet to food that hasn't been heated above 115 degrees. The theory (which I consider well-founded) is that cooking depletes food of at least 30% of its natural nutrients and all of its enzymes. Some even argue that cooking food can chemically alter its structure and may convert certain foods to toxins, carcinogens, mutagens, and free-radicals, all of which are associated with cancer.

There's no question that cooking food alters proteins – that's actually one reason we cook meat. Cooking turns chewy, rubbery raw meat into something that breaks down pretty easily in the mouth. If the heat is high enough, it also modifies a wide range of fats and oils, turning them into toxins. It's well-established that over-grilling and charring foods introduces toxins into your body. Any food that's pasteurized, processed, or refined is off limits. That means you can't eat baked goods, pasta, store-bought juices (nearly all are pasteurized), or milk -- among other things. Why go on a raw foods diet in the first place? Because advocates believe cooking reduces or eliminates the vitamins and antioxidants in foods, they contend you'll get higher levels of both if you follow the diet. So on the surface, a raw foods diet makes a lot of sense.

For starters, you wind up eating loads of fresh fruits, berries, vegetables, and nuts in their natural state. Because the food doesn't get cooked or irradiated and isn't exposed to genetic engineering or pesticides, you're all but guaranteed a higher nutritional content. A significant factor is that you're consuming thousands of plant compounds that either haven't been identified yet, or whose benefits haven't been analyzed yet. I have little doubt some of these unknown compounds pack a powerful nutritional punch.

Consider that resveratrol, curcumin, pycnogenol, anthocyanins, astaxanthin, lutein and many other familiar nutrients were unknown just a few years ago. Very likely they're just the tip of the iceberg. You're getting all those unknown wonder nutrients with a raw food diet instead of just one or two that have been isolated, extracted and put into a pill. And you're getting them in a more bioavailable form.

The raw food diet is also an effective weight-loss diet, if that's your angle. Most people who follow a raw foods diet eat only half the calories they'd get with a cooked-foods diet. Among other things, the fiber fills you up so you don't have to eat so much, and the diet doesn't include addictive, binge-inducing sugar or MSG. One thing you'll find is that foods that don't get most of us excited, like a kale salad, are delicious when you're hungry and you're not allowing yourself the easy fix of carbohydrates. At the same time, few of us will down a second helping of kale salad the way we'd scarf down a second helping of mashed potatoes. On the raw foods diet, you tend to eat until you aren't hungry anymore, and then stop. That's a good thing.

The resulting weight loss often helps prevent or control diabetes. You're not eating the sugar and refined grains that bring on insulin resistance and spikes in blood sugar. Another advantage to raw food is that it helps your body reach an alkalized state, which (according to its advocates) brings on healing, weight loss, and detoxification. I'm not a big fan of the acid/alkaline theory of disease – but without question the same diet that's said to make your body alkaline is healthy anyway, on more sensible grounds.

Other claimed benefits : You'll have more energy, better digestion, clearer skin, and you'll even be lightening the toxic burden that's wrecking the planet. It's not without risks, of course. If you follow a strict raw foods diet, you're at risk of insufficient caloric intake. In women, this can lead to amenorrhea, which causes menstrual periods to stop and may contribute to uterine cancer. Best advice with raw foods "Go half way."

Going raw is already a prominent part of disease prevention The alternative cancer world is no stranger to the value of foods in their natural state. Several famous cancer-prevention protocols rely on the raw-foods approach. The best-known is probably the Gerson Therapy, which uses an organic, plant-based diet, raw juices, coffee enemas, and natural supplements. Raw foods are not the whole show.

Raw foods are also prominent in the organic juicing trend, which gives you massive boosts of raw foods all at once, without the fiber. It goes without saying that the raw foods diet includes top foods proven to help treat and prevent cancer, such as:

Green tea

Fresh vegetables such as broccoli, cauliflower, and Brussels sprouts

- Fresh fruits such as tomato and pomegranate
- Turmeric
- Medicinal mushrooms
- Fresh wheatgrass
- Probiotics and fermented foods

Raw foods: Part of the total health package

If you're looking to stay healthy and keep your body in top condition, it's a good diet to try for short stretches at a time – say, 21 days or so. You'll get ample sources of fruits and vegetables, and you're nearly guaranteed to lose weight. After 21 days, taper off, but not all the way off. On the other hand, it's a diet with a ton of rules. It takes a lot of time to prepare the foods, compared to the diet of prepared and fast foods most people are used to. You'd be wise to invest in a quality juicer, blender, and dehydrator. Not recommended for infants and children though.

Probably the best half-measure you can take is a green smoothie every day, because it tends to be a powerful antioxidant drink and involves consuming many, many servings of raw, leafy vegetables that you probably won't find tasty in other dishes. When you juice this way you do miss the fiber, but you ingest a mega-dose of nutrients – more than you would get if you ate the whole food, because the fiber fills you up. I've seen a whole package of carrots disappear into one glass of carrot juice. At the very least, balance your diet with a good daily proportion of uncooked fruits and vegetables. It'll help reduce your toxic load and give your body ample nutrition.

The power of green tea

Matcha is a specific form of green tea that hails from Japan, unique because the tea leaves are stoneground into powder. Because of the grinding process, drinking matcha gives you much the same health benefits you'd enjoy if you actually ate a whole green tea leaf. The powder dissolves and you consume it, while with conventional tea you consume the chemical compounds released by the leaf when it's exposed to hot water – and throw the rest of the leaf away. Thus, when you drink matcha you get 100% of the nutrients from that leaf. For comparison, one cup of matcha tea is said to equal 10 cups of regularly brewed green tea.

In an antioxidant analysis of matcha green tea conducted by Brunswick Laboratories, an independent bioanalytical testing & research center in Massachusetts, matcha tea ORAC levels (oxygen radical absorbance capacity) registered at an impressive 1,573 units per gram. ORAC is the accepted measure of antioxidant power. In contrast, goji berries provide only 253 units per gram. Blueberries, acai berries, broccoli, and spinach all come in at less than 100 units per gram.

As you know, antioxidants are your body's key defense agents that help prevent chronic disease and even slow down aging. The USDA recommends you consume 5,000 ORAC units per day. A single serving of matcha (two grams) contains 2,400 ORAC units (which are also fiber-filled and sugar free). The chlorophyll content is another reason matcha green tea is superior to traditional brewed green teas. Chlorophyll is the key ingredient that lends color to matcha tea. In fact, matcha is typically grown in the shade, and because of that it tends to be richer in chlorophyll than other green teas. Chlorophyll has the added benefit of being a detoxifier. To get the deep, rich green of chlorophyll, matcha growers cover the plants with heavy shade cloths for three weeks prior to harvest in May. This causes the new shoots to develop larger, thinner leaves. The result is a better flavor and texture.

The tea is harvested by hand, and the youngest, smallest leaves are selected for the highest quality matcha. Leaves are briefly steamed to stop fermentation, then dried and packed in bales for cold storage. Six months of aging deepens the flavor to peak levels.

An antioxidant powerhouse of cancer-fighting catechins

Consuming matcha in any form gives you a greater antioxidant boost than you'd get from consuming other types of green tea. Aside from ORAC and chlorophyll levels, much of the matcha fanfare began when researchers from the University of Colorado published a study in the Journal of Chromatography A. They found that the concentration of EGCG (epigallocatechin gallate) was 137 times stronger than the amount of EGCG found in other forms of green tea. In fact, EGCG levels were also at least three times higher than the highest published value for other green teas. Remarkably, more than 60% of the catechins in matcha are EGCG.

EGCG is a catechin shown to have great potential to improve human health and fight disease. Catechins are a potent class of antioxidants found only in tea, various vegetables, nuts, and carob powder. EGCG has demonstrated potent cancer-fighting properties, including the ability to suppress tumors. It helps neutralize the effects of free radicals that attack the body through pollution, chemicals, radiation, and even UV rays – all of which can lead to cell damage associated with cancer.

EGCG has also been shown to suppress inflammation and aggressive estrogen mediators in breast tissue and can cause breast cancer cells to die. And it appears to suppress new blood flow that feeds breast cancer tumors, prevents DNA damage, and suppresses the production of breast cancer stem cells. According to Dr. Kristi Pado Funk of the Pink Lotus Breast Center in Beverly Hills, California, "Three cups of green tea a day decreases breast cancer risk by half." You can achieve the same result by drinking a single cup of matcha -- and not only do you get your three cups in, you also get seven bonus cups. The power of matcha doesn't stop there.

Matcha offers even more benefits than those just described. It's considered an excellent energy booster, yet doesn't leave you with a case of the jitters. Many matcha tea drinkers report a steady boost in energy throughout their day, as opposed to the rollercoaster effect of most caffeine drinks. Researchers at first believed this was due to matcha's caffeine content, but they have since changed their minds and believe it's the combination of matcha's natural properties. The caffeine molecules in matcha bind to larger and more stable molecules (particularly those catechins). This means the caffeine is released over time instead of all at once, unlike the typical reaction with coffee or espresso. The timed-release factor inhibits any sudden insulin increases, so you don't get the crash associated with quick drops in blood sugar that commonly affect coffee drinkers. One study even found that matcha improved physical endurance by 24%.

Evidence suggests the antioxidants in matcha can protect

against many kinds of cancer, including breast, skin, lung, stomach, prostate, ovarian, and colon cancers. But it offers still more health benefits: Matcha is high in fiber and reduces harmful cholesterol in the blood. It contains five times more L-theanine than standard green teas. L-theanine is an amino acid that creates alpha waves in the brain and helps with relaxation. Matcha also provides trace minerals and vitamins including A, B-complex, C, E, and K. It can slow the aging process thanks to the high level of antioxidants. Matcha stabilizes blood sugar levels and helps boost metabolism. Matcha supports joint health and reduces inflammation, preventing cartilage breakdown. The flavonoids in matcha tea help prevent arterial blockage, thus helping prevent cardiovascular disease. And, matcha has practically zero calories.

An easy way to clean up your free radical load

If you decide to add matcha to your diet, you may find it smells a lot like freshly mown grass. The scent may not be for everybody, but it's not hard to add flavor if it doesn't appeal to you. You can get matcha green tea from your local nutrition shop or even order it on Amazon. You won't find it in tea bags, only in powder form. Tea bags would defeat the idea of dissolving the whole leaf and consuming it.

Matcha is strong, so you really only need about one-half teaspoon per serving. Most people mix the powder with two ounces of hot water and whisk vigorously. You can then add more water, milk, or almond milk. You're best off drinking it right away or the matcha will settle to the bottom in a paste. Some people drink it straight; others prefer to add honey, agave, or a sprinkle of cocoa powder. A daily regimen of matcha tea will help restore your body's well-being and clean up your free radical load.

Now, thanks to the growing power of alternative medicine, blended and flavored green tea products have appeared on the market in mass quantities. Green tea has received a big push from natural health advocates because it's effective against multiple cancers, including esophagus, stomach, colon, bladder, prostate, ovaries, uterus, and breast. In fact, tea drinkers have up to a 68% lower risk of cancer in and around the digestive tract. Green tea has been shown to lower lung cancer risk (even for smokers!). In addition, it lowers the risk of leukemia and non-Hodgkin's lymphoma. In fact, green tea might be the best choice for the #1 beverage you should drink to fight cancer. And if you want to get the most bang for your buck, there's a particular type of green tea you need to know about. Part of the power of green tea lies in its potent antioxidant and polyphenol levels. And that's where matcha tea enters the picture and earns even more accolades – because it has even higher levels of antioxidants and other health properties.

How matcha kills cancer cells

Matcha has earned such a strong reputation in the health world that some call it a "miracle food." Given all the ways it can treat or prevent disease, that's hardly an overstatement. Take a look at some research out of the University of Salford in Manchester, England. Using metabolic phenotyping, a scientific process that examines how compounds directly impact cells, the researchers tested matcha green tea powder on breast cancer cell lines. They discovered that matcha moved the cancer cells "towards a quiescent metabolic state," which effectively stopped their proliferation. The researchers also found the cancer stem cell signaling pathways that normally promote growth were affected, appearing weaker overall.

The matcha tea extract suppresses the metabolism of cancer cells' mitochondria, the "batteries" that power the cells. Thanks to matcha's metabolic phenotyping, scientists now understand how matcha can suppress oxidative mitochondrial metabolism, a fancy way of saying that it keeps cells from "re-fueling" (meaning they become inactive and die). One of the study authors, Dr. Michael Lisanti, even said, "The effects on human breast cancer cells were very striking; the active ingredients in matcha have a surgical effect in knocking out certain signaling pathways." The experiments were conducted on breast cancer cells grown in lab cultures. We already have plenty of other evidence for the impact of green tea on cancer rates.

Don't get sidetracked by green fads

If you decide to add matcha to your diet, make sure you get the real thing – that is, the tea powder. Thanks to the consumer craze that has followed this potent green substance, you can now get matcha-dyed soba noodles, matcha mochi, matcha lattes, and even matcha green tea ice cream. These faddish foods might be better than nothing, but none of them will ever give you as many nutrients as a solid cup of matcha tea. If you're taking green tea supplements, don't overdo them. Even when a nutrient is beneficial, sometimes too much of it can be toxic. So drink the tea, preferably in the matcha version.

Pineapple, bromelain and raw foods

A natural enzyme that's been proven safer and more effective than a blockbuster chemotherapy drug that oncologists have been pushing at patients for 40 years. In an animal study, researchers discovered that an enzyme called bromelain, contained in pineapple stems, was a better cancer treatment than the chemotherapy agent 5-fluorauracil. The study was published in the journal Planta Medica. Researchers stated, "This antitumoral effect [of bromelain] was superior to that of 5-FU [5-fluorouracil]..."

What makes this result particularly impressive is that bromelain caused no harm to the animals. So the pineapple plant not only yields a favorite fruit, but also a powerful medicine. Compare gentle but powerful bromelain to the grim track record of 5-FU, a drug in which millions of cancer patients have placed their hope of recovery for the past 40 years – and a drug they've paid billions of dollars to obtain. 5-FU is unaffectionately known as "five feet under" because, like most chemo, it doesn't work very well. It is unable to kill only cancer cells, and often kills or irreversibly damages healthy cells and tissue as well.

GreenMedInfo observes:

"As a highly toxic, fluoride-bound form of the nucleic acid uracil, a normal component of RNA, the drug is supposed to work by tricking more rapidly dividing cells – which include both cancer and healthy intestinal, hair follicle, and immune cells – into taking it up, thereby inhibiting (read: poisoning) RNA-replication enzymes and RNA synthesis...

"...When a person dies following conventional cancer treatment it is all too easy to 'blame the victim' and simply write that patient's cancer off as 'chemo-resistant,' or 'exceptionally aggressive,' when in fact the non-selective nature [damage to healthy cells] of the chemotoxic agent is what ultimately led to their death."

Its safety data sheets calls 5-FU "very hazardous" You might want to take a hint from the Material Safety Data Sheet (MSDS) for 5-FU. It warns about the substance's deadly nature. Potential Acute Health Effects:

"Very hazardous in case of skin contact (irritant), of ingestion. Hazardous in case of inhalation. Slightly hazardous in case of skin contact (permeator), or eye contact (irritant). Severe over-exposure can result in death."

Potential Chronic Health Effects:

"... The substance is toxic to blood. Repeated or prolonged exposure to the substance can produce target organs damage. Repeated exposure to a highly toxic material may produce general deterioration of health by an accumulation in one or many human organs."

A 5-FU dosage of 115 mg per kilogram of body weight kills half of the animals that consume it – the equivalent of a 7.8

gram dosage for a 150-pound adult. That's the weight of a mere 3 pennies.

Compare this to bromelain's Medical Safety Data Sheet. The amount of bromelain that would kill 50% of adults is 1.5 pounds of bromelain. That means the pineapple enzyme is approximately 87 times safer than 5-FU. Some sources even say it's three orders of magnitudes safer! The history of 5-FU is a picture of arrogant modern science gone horribly awry. Compare it to the life-giving history of the pineapple.

Christopher Columbus became the first European to learn about pineapples, on the island of Guadeloupe in 1493. He took this South American treasure back to Europe as one of his most exotic prizes from the New World. I'm not sure if he knew about its medicinal qualities, as opposed to its delicious taste. But native populations in South America have used pineapples for hundreds of years to quell inflammation and infections. By the 1600s, pineapples were very popular in Europe.

In colonial America, sailors brought pineapples home to New England. A fresh pineapple displayed on the front porch meant the sailor had returned from foreign ports and was ready to receive visitors. The pineapple is still a symbol of welcome, at least in parts of the eastern United States where people are mindful of tradition. This exotic fruit was considered the height of elegance, and was often the crowning glory of early American banquets. George Washington grew pineapples in the hothouse on his property. If conventional doctors were open to natural cancer treatments, they'd sit up and take notice of the amazing enzyme contained in this fruit.

How bromelain works

Indigenous cultures knew that bromelain was useful for fighting inflammation. Cancer – like many other conditions – is actually linked to chronic inflammation in your body. The only question is whether inflammation causes cancer, or is a byproduct of cancer – or both. Few people know this, but you don't actually get much bromelain from eating the most popular part of the fruit. Only small quantities of the enzyme are found in the juice of the pineapple. The most potent cancer-fighting properties are found in the pineapple's core.

Ironically, that's the part most people toss in the trash. Instead of throwing it away because it's pulpy, you can juice it and feast on its cancer-fighting powers. When you do, you'll reap one of the most prized benefits of natural cancer treatments. "Selective cytotoxicity" is a well-known property of many natural compounds. In layman's terms, that means a substance kills only cancer cells, without killing healthy cells – and you.

No FDA-approved chemotherapy drug on the market can claim this priceless benefit. That's one reason today's conventional cancer treatment methods are still in the Dark Ages – at best, destroying quality of life, and at worst, causing death. You and I both know bromelain will never receive FDA approval as a cancer treatment even if it works, because non-patentable substances don't result in big paydays for pharmaceutical companies. And bromelain isn't the only compound that offers selective cytotoxicity. Many natural foods do.

Dissolves the cloak that hides cancer cells

Bromelain is a proteolytic enzyme (meaning it digests proteins). Such enzymes are also called proteases. Proteolytic enzymes can help fight cancer by:

• Decreasing inflammation.

• Boosting cytokines, especially interferon and tumor necrosis factor, which are critical warriors in the fight against cancer cells.

• Dissolving fibrin, the cloak behind which cancer cells hide to escape detection. Once they're "uncloaked," your immune system can attack and destroy them. Researchers also think fibrin lets cancer cells stick together, allowing them to metastasize.

• Boosting the potency of the immune system's macrophages and killer cells 12-fold, according to German studies.

However, getting enzymes from your digestive tract into your bloodstream may be more challenging than you think. In the Planta Medica study described at the beginning of this article, in which bromelain outperformed 5-FU, the natural enzyme was injected directly into the abdominal cavity.

Don't make this mistake with supplemental bromelain

The use of supplemental enzymes is becoming more popular in the U.S. But its roots go back more than 100 years to John Beard's 1911 book, The Enzyme Treatment of Cancer and Its Scientific Basis. New York City Doctor Nick Gonzalez, an MD, has also written a book on using enzymes for cancer treatment. In fact, treating cancer with proteolytic enzymes of all kinds has a long pedigree and is one of the most popular alternative treatments.

Bromelain is just the tip of the iceberg. There's a whole array of enzymes boasting a host of health benefits. They are among the best and safest anti-inflammatories – an ideal natural pain remedy. When using proteolytic enzymes to treat cancer, alternative doctors say you shouldn't take them with food, because they'll act as digestive enzymes, and won't work throughout your entire system. To get system-wide benefits, take them without food. Generally, it's also recommended that a cancer patient take very large amounts of proteolytic enzymes. There's a more pleasant approach than taking huge numbers of enzyme pills: raw foods.

Raw foods are the most potent natural source of enzymes. In their unprocessed state, fruits and vegetables are rich in these nutrients. In contrast, cooked and processed foods, whether organic or not, contain few enzymes because heat destroys or denatures these long, complex molecules. If we all ate enough raw foods we might not need the supplements, but in this age of processed and fast food, most people don't consume enough enzymes. Notch your health upwards by trying to fill 75 to 80 percent of your daily diet with raw organic foods – these contain plenty of enzymes and fewer pesticides and herbicides. Juicing your vegetables and pineapple cores is a good way to increase the amount of nutrients and enzymes entering your system.

Whole raw foods are better than pills for another reason: Besides enzymes they contain a whole treasure house of other nutrients you won't find in pills. Many of these nutrients haven't even been identified, named and studied yet. That means new ones are being discovered all the time. But don't wait for a journal article to come out. You can reap the benefits of these unknown nutrients now – just by eating raw, unprocessed foods. The more raw foods you eat, the more enzymes and other phytonutrients you provide for healthy internal functions – from digestion to fighting cancer, and many things in between. And the more enzymes you have – in excess of what you need to digest your food -- the better these nutrients can perform the other health and regenerative functions you need.

Another herb for the prostate

Deadly nightshade is one of the most toxic plants, causing delirium, hallucinations, convulsions and possibly death to the unlucky soul who eats enough of it. Unfortunately, another plant is often confused with deadly nightshade, yet is not only edible and nutritious, but acts against cancer in many ways. It's called black nightshade. Black nightshade (Solanum nigrum) is part of a family of plants that includes tomatoes, chili peppers, egg plants and potatoes. All of these relatives of black nightshade are sometimes grouped together as the nightshade vegetables. Dozens of related plants used to be grouped together under S.nigrum – they were all called black nightshade -- but many are now being reclassified as separate species. S. nigrum is native to Europe and the Mediterranean and is often called European black nightshade.

In the US, S. ptychanthum dominates in the East, and S.

americanum dominates in the South. The Great Plains is home to S. interius, and S. douglasii is found in the Southwest. Sometimes the whole group is referred to as Solanum nigrum complex. Other names for black nightshade are Duscle, Garden Nightshade, Hound's Berry, Petty Morel, and Wonder Berry. Unlike deadly nightshade, where the berries grow individually, black nightshade berries grow in bunches. They start out green, then ripen to dark purple-black berries ready to pick in the late summer and fall. They're safe to eat.

The flavor is said to be sweet with a savory hint, like a cross between a tomato, a tomatillo and a blueberry (Warning: if the berry hasn't fully ripened and doesn't taste sweet, do not eat it). Although the ripe berries and leaves are consumed by up to a quarter of the world's population, the plant is widely believed to be toxic, probably because of its historic confusion with deadly nightshade (Atropa belladonna).

Nicholas Culpeper, in his Complete Herbal, first published in 1653, wrote, "Have a care you mistake not the deadly nightshade for this [black nightshade]; if you know it not, then you may let them both alone." Modern day wild plant authority and author Samuel Thayer assures us, "Through an extensive search of literary sources and consultation with experts, I have been unable to locate a single, credible, documented case of poisoning from the ripe berries of any member of the S. nigrum complex.

The European species of black nightshades were known to the ancient Greeks and Romans, who used them medicinally. In the 1st century AD, Pliny the Elder documented its use against stings, wounds and lumbago (lower back pain). In traditional Indian (Ayurveda) medicine, black nightshade infusions are used to relieve fever, stomach complaints and dysentery. The juice is used to treat ulcers and skin diseases. The fruit or leaves are used for asthma, tuberculosis, whooping cough, and liver diseases.

The plant is also part of traditional Chinese medicine,

where practitioners believe it acts as an antioxidant and diuretic, possesses anti-inflammatory, liver protective, and anti-fever properties, and can relieve mastitis (a breast tissue infection). Black nightshade is also frequently included in cancer therapy. Medicinal uses in Africa include antiseptic for eyes and skin, treatment of diarrhea, and as a general tonic for health.

It's quite a grab bag of medical claims, and we don't have sufficient evidence for all of these traditional uses. Laboratory studies support some of them. Four rodent studies have tested its effects on the liver and found it protected against scarring (fibrosis), alcoholic liver damage, paracetamol-induced toxicity, and poisoning by cadmium chloride. Other studies have found black nightshade protects the brain from free radicals generated by physical or psychological stress and has anti-fungal, anti-allergy, anti-inflammatory and anti-convulsant effects. That particular group of benefits suggests black nightshade is some kind of antioxidant, and further evidence confirms a much.

Suppresses tumor growth

In 2003, South Korean researchers carried out an early study that looked into Solanum nigrum as a potential anti-cancer agent. They prepared an extract from ripe fruit and tested it on human breast cancer cells grown in a lab culture. It turned out the extract "strongly suppressed" the ability of the cells to grow, and it did so by inducing apoptosis (cancer cell suicide). The researchers also found it was a good scavenger of free radicals. They concluded that the "extract could be used as an antioxidant and cancer chemo-preventive material." The following year, another research group from South Korea tested a different extract from the plant on human colon cancer cells.

Again, they found it was toxic to these cells and induced apoptosis by inhibiting various proteins that are involved with the promotion of tumors. They speculated that the extract "could be used as a chemotherapy agent even at low concentrations." Since then there have been over 50 research papers looking at the effect of different extracts of S. nigrum on cancer cells lines.

Anti-tumor effects have been found for leukemia, prostate, liver, bile duct, lung, stomach, bladder, pancreas, skin (melanoma), endometrial and cervical cancer through many different cellular pathways and by activation of apoptosis and autophagy. Autophagy is a cellular process by which misfolded proteins and other cellular debris that could damage the cell are swept away, protecting the cell and promoting its survival.

Reduces tumor weight and volume

Recent studies have looked to mice experiments for confirmation of these in vitro (cell culture) findings. Two studies were published in 2016. In the first, scientists from Taiwan tested two extracts of S. nigrum on tumor-bearing mice. Both extracts significantly reduced the volume and weight of the tumors, as well as the expression of CD31, a marker for angiogenesis - growth of the blood supply to the tumor. In addition, the black nightshade extracts inhibited vascular endothelial growth factor (VEGF), which helps feed angiogenesis.

In a further experiment they found human liver cancer cells were inhibited by both extracts and this was correlated with inhibition of AKT/mTOR, an intracellular signaling pathway important in the regulation of the cell cycle. In the second study, Malaysian scientists fed a polysaccharide fraction from S. nigrum to mice with breast tumors for ten days. The treatment inhibited tumor volume by a significant 65% and tumor weight by 40%. Analysis of blood, tumor, spleen, and thymus found an increase in certain immune cells in the tumor tissue and higher apoptosis in the treated mice. The researchers concluded that tumor suppression came about through boosting immune response. This is in line with previous research which showed the same extract modulated the immune system.

Shrank tumors in this mice study

The most recent study was published in the Journal of Cancer Research and Therapeutics in 2018. Here the scientists also looked at the effect of a polysaccharide fraction in mice with liver cancer. They were particularly interested in the expression of caspase-3, a protein which induces apoptosis (cancer cell death), and bcl-2, a family of proteins that can act as a barrier to apoptosis and facilitate tumor development and resistance to cancer therapy. Mice were given three different concentrations of S. nigrum polysaccharides daily for ten days.

The black nightshade extract reduced the average tumor weight compared to the control group. The tumor inhibition rates were 37.73%, 38.24%, and 42.60%, with rates rising as the dose increased. The protein expression of caspase-3 (inducing cancer cell death) in S. nigrum groups was higher, but the expression of bcl-2 (prevents cancer cell death) was lower than the control group in a dose-dependent manner. Other tests indicated an improvement in immune function. The researchers wrote that black nightshade "possesses obvious cytotoxicity to the tumor and inhibits tumor cell growth."

All research on black nightshade has been carried out in Asian countries. The only exception was a study by Case Western Reserve University, Cleveland, Ohio. They wrote: "Our results, for the first time, demonstrate that the S. nigrum extract is capable of selectively inhibiting cellular proliferation and accelerating apoptotic events in prostate cancer cells. S. nigrum may be developed as a promising therapeutic and/or preventive agent against prostate cancer." You will see a nod to beneficial effects of the toxin in nightshade, yet taken in a far more safer way with an equivalent remedy in my earlier chapter on homeopathy.

Keeping out the poop

A medical study recently has confirmed what you may have always suspected: that most people are full of ... well, poop. In a study of autopsies, examiners found that 90% of the cadavers' colons held an average of 5 to 20 pounds of hardened, decayed feces which were encrusted in layers on the intestine walls. Extrapolating this on the living population, it means that a staggering number of adults (including you) are walking around with a backed-up bowel that holds pounds of old, impacted feces that is protruding their bellies and secretly making them ill, besides messing up their probiotics. Whew!

This was confirmed by a European medical study which found that a whopping 62% of adults whom doctors examined had an average of 10-12 pounds of residual fecal matter buildup in their large intestines and rectums. Obviously, the majority of people today are not completely emptying their bowels of noxious waste products everyday as nature intended. But when the doctors gave these poor people a treatment of a special all-natural colon-cleansing substance, their bowel mass was reduced from 42% to 17%. This is an amazing reduction!

Not only were they able to completely empty their bowels, but this re-established their natural bowel rhythm so they remained "clean and regular" afterward. In addition to much easier bowel movements, the patients reported feeling thinner, lighter, healthier and more energized. Their stomachs were happy too! This is where probiotics help and help tremendously restore a healthy gut and energized body. Your gut bacteria army is an important player in supporting detoxification through poop removal. This regular detoxification with your trillions strong internal army is yet another arrow in your powerful quiver against cancer. It follows naturally from healthy eating, avoiding processed foods and artificial additives, that we have already emphasized earlier in the book.

Rest and timing

Round the clock stimulation from screens and the light they emit. Late night TV. Inadequate amounts of sleep. Snacking at all hours. These and other lifestyle factors disrupt ancient, deeply ingrained biological processes -- our internal body clocks and the circadian rhythms they control. This disruption has been linked to diseases ranging from Alzheimer's to ulcerative colitis. Cancer is among them.

You can restore your body's natural rhythms and boost your health with a few simple lifestyle changes. Yes, you need to turn out the lights, turn off the screens, and go to bed at a reasonable hour. You don't have to fly across several times zones to get jet lag. Nearly nine out of ten of us suffer from social jet lag, a condition caused by living a lifestyle that's out of synch with our natural sleep-wake cycle. Scientists have found that virtually every aspect of our life is rhythmic, and we are programmed to go through specific rhythms on a daily basis. This internal timing system, called the circadian rhythm, interacts with the times of day when light enters our eyes, and even the times of day when we eat, to create our daily rhythms.

To everything there is a time

Humans were around for a few hundred thousand years before there were light bulbs, not to mention screens. When it's dark our bodies are programmed to be asleep, and when the sun rises we're supposed to be up and around. Since the body would be overwhelmed if it carried out all its activities at once, each one has a specific time. This allows biological functions to be optimized. For instance, before we wake up, the sleep hormone melatonin starts to shut down, while breathing, heart beat and blood pressure pick up a little. During daylight, immune response improves and muscles are primed for activity. After dark a whole range of other activities either kick in or slow down.

Melatonin – the "sleep hormone" – is at a low point first thing in the morning and builds steadily during the day to reach a peak when it's bedtime. Our energy or wakefulness hormone, cortisol, has the opposite cycle. Cortisol is a low point when we go to bed, and its level rises steadily through the night to reach a peak in the morning. Exposure to light in the middle of the night or to darkness during the day disrupts this natural process." While circadian rhythms are influenced by light, the timing they follow is under the control of genes. Every single gene in our genome has a circadian cycle, with thousands turning on and off at different times in different organs in a synchronized manner to optimize cell function. Cellular energy, maintenance, repair, division, secretion and communication all occur in a cyclical manner.

Your body's master clock

Standing at the summit of this process is the suprachiasmatic nucleus (SCN), a small cluster of cells located in the brain's hypothalamus that act as the master clock. It receives information that morning light has entered the eyes and shares it with the liver clock, the heart clock, the gut clock and every other clock in the body. These organs then create their own circadian rhythms. The SCN is also connected to the hunger center in the brain.

Among the variety of circadian rhythms, there are three that stand out. These are related to when you eat, when and how much you sleep, and when and how often you engage in physical activity. Fortunately, all three are under our control, although in the real world – the modern one we live in -- optimizing the timing of these activities may be hard to achieve depending on people's domestic, work and travel schedules. We'll come back to the most favorable timing of meals, sleep and exercise in a minute.

Shift workers have weaker immune systems

Like all our organs, the immune system has a circadian component, and disruptions to our core rhythms will cause it to function less well, making us more susceptible to infections and disease, and slowing recovery from illness. People who have to work the night shift experience a profound disruption in their relation to natural light, meals and sleep. Studies show they have much more fragile immune systems. They not only have a higher cancer rate, but they're also more prone to bacterial infections, gastric and duodenal ulcers, inflammatory bowel disease, cardiovascular disease, and arthritis. In 2007, The International Agency for Research on Cancer declared shift work to be "probably carcinogenic" and several large studies have linked this disruption to various cancers.

Night workers suffer more breast, prostate cancer

The Fred Hutchinson Cancer Research Center in Seattle found that "Graveyard shiftwork was associated with increased breast cancer risk with a trend of increased risk with increasing years and with more hours per week of graveyard shiftwork." A separate study found nurses on long-term rotating night shifts had a marked increase in the risk of breast cancer. Similar findings were obtained for prostate cancer risk in night shift workers.

In a 30-year study of 161,000 women, those who worked a rotating schedule had a 27% increased risk of fatal ovarian cancer compared to those on fixed daytime work. Researchers from the Dana-Farber Cancer Institute and Brigham and Women's Hospital in Boston found that "Women working rotating night shifts for a long duration have a significantly increased risk of endometrial cancer." Another group from Brigham and Women's and Harvard found that nurses working a rotating night shift at least three nights a month for 15 or more years had a significantly increased risk of colorectal cancer. Laboratory research in rodents supports human studies. Circadian disruption kicks off the cancer process and increases tumor growth.

How a disrupted body clock disrupts your health

A malfunctioning internal clock causes immune imbalance, where some types of immune cell are overproduced while others are deficient. The circadian clock also regulates basic defense mechanisms within all cells such as the control of oxidative stress (free radicals). It acts as a sensor for excess free radicals and co-ordinates antioxidant defense mechanisms. Autophagy, the process by which cellular garbage is disposed of or recycled, is also regulated by a clock.

If oxidative stress is not controlled and the autophagy system is under par, the body can resort to an emergency defense system to neutralize cellular damage and stress, but this causes chronic inflammation and compromises other essential body functions. A mouse study found that when a protein that's a core clock component was removed, every cell behaved as if it was under attack and produced a state of chronic inflammation.

Shortens telomeres – and your life

A body clock that's out of sync not only increases oxidative stress, limits autophagy and promotes inflammation, but has other negative consequences. It reduces the length of telomeres, found at the end of chromosomes. This has been shown to increase the risk of breast cancer – and, in general, shorter telomeres correlate with a reduced life span. When the body's clock is off, immune system surveillance becomes compromised, allowing cancer cells to escape and grow to form tumors. Metabolism speeds up, too. This fuels cancer growth.

There's more: the body loses some of its ability to repair DNA damage, which increases the chances of developing cancer. Since many cancer-related cellular processes -- the cell cycle, cell proliferation, cell suicide (apoptosis), DNA damage -- are influenced by the circadian clock, you'd expect disruption to this system, such as found in shift workers, to have detrimental effects.

Medications work better when the timing is right

Patients' ability to tolerate nearly 500 medications was shown to improve by as much as fivefold when matched to the circadian system. This also applies to chemotherapy. The first study to demonstrate this -- over 30 years ago -- found mistiming drugs led to much more severe chemo side effects. This has been confirmed in many other studies. The same probably applies to surgery as well. A mouse study found regrowth of the liver differed considerably depending on whether the surgery took place in the morning or afternoon.

Mice given total body irradiation in the morning lost 80% of their hair. Others undergoing the same procedure in the evening lost only 20% of their hair. Because tumors have poorly functioning clocks, scientists recently came up with the idea to develop drugs that bind to clock molecules to restore healthy function. In 2017, Canadian scientists found that clock gene expression could be restored in melanoma cells and tumors. Glioblastoma (brain cancer) cells implanted into mice grew aggressively. But other mice receiving a "clock-modifying drug" saw remarkably reduced tumor growth and survived longer. The clock drug was more effective than the standard drug used to treat brain cancer.

Change your daily routine

Our physiology is largely the same as it was in our ancestors two million years ago, so our internal clocks are out of sync with the society we live in today. If we want a strong immune system and a reduced risk of cancer and other health problems, we need to make a few lifestyle tweaks to send us back a little in time. Professor Satchin Panda, a leading expert in the field of circadian rhythm research at the Salk Institute in San Diego, writes in his book The Circadian Code that "to have predictable circadian rhythms is to have healthy organs" and that "repeatedly disrupting your circadian clock can have adverse health consequences, as every system in your body starts to malfunction."

To bring circadian rhythms back into line he suggests the following:

Sleep: Go to bed around 10 PM or so and aim for seven to eight hours consecutive sleep. The brain takes many minutes to unwind, so shut off all devices well before bedtime and limit or dim artificial light as much as possible during the evening. Bedroom temperature should be 70° or lower. Wake up naturally, without the help of an alarm clock, and get some bright light immediately after waking. Follow this pattern every day including weekends. Personally, I find I don't need an alarm. I set one to be safe, but I always wake up before it goes off.

Exercise: When not eating or sleeping the body was designed for movement, so keep active, move as much as you can, and only sit for short periods at a time. Physical activity also improves sleep. Our ancestors were active all day but especially early morning and late afternoon/early evening, so these are preferred times. Exercise outdoors and soak up the light for best results. If you exercise indoors, do it by a window.

Fix your sleep routine. Your body will thank you. It will also help fight cancer more naturally using its own in-built detox system that operates while you sleep.

Super Vitamin D

D3 deficiency has serious consequences for good health. The vast majority of the population is deficient, and there's reason to believe it underlies a wide range of major health problems. So how do you know if you're deficient? The following symptoms are signals and should be brought to your doctor's IMMEDIATE attention:

1. Bone Loss:

A diagnosis of low bone mineral density may be a major sign of vitamin D deficiency. Getting enough of this vitamin is important for preserving bone mass as you get older. Many older women who are diagnosed with bonc loss believe they need to take more calcium. However, they may be deficient in vitamin D as well.

2. Getting Sick or Infected Often:

One of vitamin D's most important roles is keeping your

immune system strong so you're able to fight off the viruses and bacteria that cause illness. Vitamin D plays an important role in immune function.

3. Chronic Fatigue and Tiredness

Feeling tired can have many causes and vitamin D deficiency may be one of them. In one case, a woman who complained of chronic daytime fatigue and headaches was found to have a D3 blood level of only 5.9 ng/ml. (Anything under 20 ng/ml is deficient). When the woman took a vitamin D supplement, her level increased to 39 ng/ml and her symptoms resolved.

4. Bone and Back Pain:

Bone pain and lower back pain may be signs of inadequate vitamin D levels in the blood. Vitamin D is involved in maintaining bone health through a number of mechanisms. For one, it improves your body's absorption of calcium. People with vitamin D deficiency are nearly twice as likely to experience bone pain in their legs or joints compared to those with blood levels in the normal range.

5. Depression:

A depressed mood may also be a sign of deficiency. In review studies, researchers have linked vitamin D deficiency to depression, particularly in older adults. Some studies have found supplementing with D improves mood. When you notice persistent health issues like these, you may want to consider a quality Vitamin D3 + Vitamin K2 supplement.

We also talked of the VDRTaq SNP that can be uncovered in genetic tests discussed in previous chapters. This will another reason to supplement if you have the SNP, once you have verified that your Vitamin D levels are indeed low. Use a doctor's advice if taking higher doses of Vitamin D as it is fat soluble and tends to accumulate in the body like Vitamin A.

Exercise the second

A lot of us know what we need to do to secure good health and stave off diseases like cancer. We all know we need to eat right, exercise, reduce stress, practice gratitude. But actually doing those things can be tough. Not only do you have to make time for good choices, you also need the willpower to get out there and make it happen. So it's worth discussing some trusted techniques for summoning the willpower we all need to develop so we can stick to good health habits. For someone who does not like exercise, this could be a battle by itself.

Human to the core

Our willpower is only as strong, and sometimes not as strong as, our human needs. The man who eats cake when offered isn't a bad person, nor is he weak. He's just hungry. Really, it's a brain thing. The concept of willpower is just a tug-of-war between logical conclusions you worked out in your prefrontal cortex – what you know you should do – matched in a smackdown against the power-pull of your primal appetites and emotions.

As it turns out, willpower is a finite resource. We only have so much of it. According to social psychologist Roy Baumeister, any act of resisting temptation (like that cake) leaves you less capable of resisting anything else you're trying to power past, or any difficult choice you have to make. And that's just average, daily temptation for the average person on a normal day. When you're battling a serious disease like cancer or facing the emotional toll of watching a friend or family member fight through it, your energy reserves – including willpower – are even further depleted.

Who among us doesn't reach for comfort foods when we've had a bad day? And then the depleted willpower leads to more weak moments and bad decisions. It affects what you eat, what you think, and whether you engage in any positive health behaviors like exercise, meditation, or even laughing with friends.

Identify your "strong hour"

Everybody has a "strong" hour during the day when willpower is highest and the ability to make good decisions is strongest. For most people, it occurs in the morning, after a solid night's sleep. Though there are exceptions, such as people who feel best following a midday nap or those who find their energy levels soar in the evenings. The first step in bolstering willpower is to identify your "strong time" and alter your schedule so you tackle your biggest challenges then. If getting to the gym or sitting down to meditate is a stumbling block, set up your day so you do that hard thing when you're feeling your strongest. And then do it.

There's an additional upside here. If you go ahead and do the hardest thing you have trouble getting motivated to do, then – guess what – you've just scored a win! Meaning, if you know you've already done that one hard thing you haven't been able to get to for weeks, and you still have hours left in the day, you'll be that much stronger when you go on to make other willpower-based decisions. Whereas a failure further lessens your willpower, a win makes it stronger. And it just builds from there, in whichever direction you've started your day. A lot of emphasis is placed on strengthening the will. It's like a muscle. You work it out, it gets stronger.

6 Simple strategies to boost your willpower

There are several other proven techniques for bolstering willpower and keeping up motivation. For example:

• Purge temptations. If junk food is your weak spot, get it out of the house. You'll be healthier for not having it around, and you won't be faced with a continual onslaught of enticements that detract from good health. I don't have sweets in the house. When I get the yen, they just aren't there, and I'm not going out to a store. I'm not that much of an addict.

• Distract and bribe. If you have the impulse to binge or drink or eat something you're trying to avoid, try the "if—then" technique. This is where you make the agreement to do the thing you really want to do – like head out to a fast food joint for a burger, but only if you first follow through on a healthy behavior, like 30 minutes on the exercise bike or writing a page in a gratitude journal. More often than not, the healthy behavior will heighten your confidence and commitment to health so that when you're done, you won't want that burger after all.

• Build an army. As anyone fighting a life-threatening disease knows, a support system plays multiple roles in keeping your spirits up and helping you past challenges. If you have a temptation you're trying to overcome, like alcohol or smoking, or if you're trying to get the hang of a smart new health behavior, like yoga, tell someone you know who supports you, and ask for their help. Being accountable to someone else and knowing they're rooting for you is an effective way to stay strong – because you have someone else holding you up.

• Get out of Dodge. Sometimes, it's our environment that's our worst enemy. Even if you have unhealthy foods purged from your environment, you may still feel enormous stress or emotional angst based on where you live, who you live with, or any number of other stressful factors. It could even be your job, your coworkers, or the level of pollution in your city. If that's the case, the best thing to do is move. Yes, it's a pain, but it can be just what you need. Even if you can't pull off a full relocation to another town, you might be able to move to another house, stay with a friend, work remotely from a new place, or switch jobs. Getting yourself out of a stressful situation that muddles your mental strength is often worth the effort it takes to make the change.

- Explore little wins. Overhauling your diet and your physical health can be a major thing, especially in our culture or if you've spent years living and eating a certain way. If you build yourself up with little wins, like waking up just five minutes earlier or forcing yourself to change a speech pattern (like dropping a habitual swear word), then little by little you'll extend your willpower.
- Forgive your humanness. You're human, and you will slip up. But giving in to one unhealthy meal or a week of not exercising is not going to doom you to a life of disease and an early death. It doesn't define who you are. Forgive any mistakes you make and move forward with the resolve to keep trying. It's all any of us can do.

So many things, from laughing more to walking outside to eating farm-fresh plant foods are proven to improve our health and bolster our immune systems against foes like cancer. But none of that does any good unless you're first able to summon the willpower it takes to do those things. Follow these six strategies until your good health behaviors become a habit. Here's hoping a long and healthy life is your reward in the end!

Can you trust Dr Google

So you're having a health problem and decide to investigate alternative options by asking "Dr. Google." Not such a great idea. What you find might be a partial or complete hoax. The website you land on may also put you at risk by denying you access to balanced, accurate information about your care options. Unfortunately, this problem isn't confined to Google. Take Wikipedia, for example.

Wiki's anti-holistic bias

Two years ago, in 2017, Wikipedia violated its own standards for neutrality by slapping acupuncture with the derogatory label of "pseudoscience" and lumping it in with astrology, Angel Healing, Reiki, and alchemy. Wikipedia's policies comprise a long spiel of legal verbiage, but my understanding is, "Articles must not take sides, but should explain the sides, fairly and without editorial bias. This applies to both what you say and how you say it." Despite this policy and an impressive body of evidence supporting acupuncture, Wiki still calls this therapy pseudoscience.

So what exactly is "supporting evidence?"

- The Joint Commission accredits more than 21,000 hospitals and health care organizations and programs worldwide. It approves acupuncture (and chiropractic, massage, physical therapy, and more) as a first-line treatment for pain.
- The Agency for Healthcare Research and Quality (AHRQ) found acupuncture to be very effective for low back pain.
- The American Academy of Family Physicians approves acupuncture for several pain conditions.
- The Joint Clinical Practice Guideline from the American College of Physicians approves the use of acupuncture, as does the American Pain Society on the Diagnosis and Treatment of Low Back Pain.
- Cochrane systematic reviews demonstrate clinical effectiveness as shown by an explosion of research on acupuncture – as a modality for headaches, osteoarthritis, fibromyalgia, cancer pain, and IBS. Cochrane Reviews are considered the gold standard for evidence in medicine.
- The National Institute for Health and Care Excellence (NICE) recommends acupuncture for prevention of migraines and tension headaches. In fact, for tension headaches, it's the only recommended treatment.
- The National Institutes of Health PubMed database contains more than 28,200 studies on acupuncture.

The US military has utilized acupuncture for well over a decade, and eight of the ten best-rated US cancer hospitals offer it onsite. Acupuncture clearly enjoys broad mainstream scientific support, in addition to boasting a 5,000-year history in Chinese Medicine. And it's pseudoscience? Really? Seems like the widespread scientific support would render Wiki's pseudoscience statement false. Acupuncture can often bring temporary relief from the health problem of the moment, whatever it may be.

How Wikipedia misleads

To support the claim that "acupuncture is pseudoscience," Wikipedia's page administrators censor the vast body of evidence that says otherwise. They regularly delete high-quality peer-reviewed systematic reviews that oppose their view, plus bully and ban comments meant to maintain neutrality. If this isn't blatant censorship, what is? Wikipedia does not permit comments on a great many articles, and it certainly doesn't permit laypeople to suggest edits. It is most certainly NOT a user-edited website. In reality, anonymous Wikipedia editors beholden to special interest groups control pages. It is it not clear who pulls the strings nor how you become a member of the inner circle that is allowed to edit and comment. And Wikipedia is not the only false, nontransparent info source.

Beware of astroturfers

Investigative journalist Sheryl Attkisson, five-time Emmy award-winning anchor, producer, and reporter, presented an excellent TEDx Talk about how Big Pharma, media, political parties, and other special interest groups propagandize you on a daily basis. The practice is called astroturfing. So what exactly is "astroturfing?" It's a false or fake "grassroots" movement. These organizations make it look like a "little guy" at the grassroots level runs them. But nothing could be further from the truth. Fake activist groups and grassroots movements are so effective, the technique has overtaken Congressional lobbying as the preferred propaganda method. As Ms. Attkisson points out, Wikipedia is an astroturfer's dream come true.

Wiki editors freely bully and banish those who present opposing views. Even factual errors are impossible to correct. In one bizarre example, Attkisson describes how the renowned novelist Philip Roth tried to correct a factual error about a character in one of his books. His correction was repeatedly reversed. He was eventually told he was not considered a credible source – about his own book.

Worse for your health, a study comparing Wikipedia's information on medical conditions with published research showed that Wikipedia contradicted the medical literature a shocking 90% of the time. Drug companies have also edited the material about side effects on Wikipedia's pages, aiming to make their drugs look more innocuous.

WebMD is no better

WebMD is one of the most visited health sites, and is generally considered a trustworthy source of "independent and objective" health information. I consult it from time to time on indications and side effects of herbal medicines, and it seems generally fair. But at times it's yet another wolf in sheep's clothing, so watch out.

Kathleen M. Zelman, MPH, RD, LD, is WebMD's director of nutrition, and has strong ties to Monsanto (now a division of Bayer). Monsanto originated Roundup weed killer and has been a driving force behind the move to GMO crops. It's the poster child for industrialized factory farming. The fact that WebMD's nutrition director is being paid by Monsanto to talk about the "wonders" of Monsanto products is alarming, to say the least. It's not likely her views are neutral.

Besides that, Monsanto is a heavy advertiser on WebMD, in some cases sponsoring "advertorials" that appear to be unbiased journalism, if you don't read the fine print. Given all this, it's not surprising that WebMD is chock-full of pro-GMO articles. To be fair, GMO foods may be safe – or at least rank low on the list of things to worry about -- but I don't think the question is fully resolved. My point here is that an objective site shouldn't employ a spokesperson for one side.

You can count out TV, radio, and print, too

Ninety percent of news media outlets are controlled by a mere handful of players. And believe me, these players have far too much to gain from running lucrative drug ads to risk having them pulled if true investigative journalism found fault with those very drugs. No wonder so many stories get pulled after they're written. Attkisson left CBS in 2015 to pursue more independent reporting. She wrote the books Stonewalled and The Smear, which reveal how these operatives work behind the scenes to promote their secret agendas.

Fake news can break your health

The manipulation and info distortion is so rife. Don't believe anything you read or see on any subject without verification from multiple sources. It doesn't matter how intelligent or scholarly or carefully footnoted the article is. We live in the golden age of "plausible narratives" and made-up facts that get repeated over and over until accepted as true. Quite often the perpetrators fervently believe their own story. Quite often the footnotes just link to other biased, partisan sources.

If you read only one side of an issue, from vaccines to what happened at the Battle of Normandy, you end up being just another one of the millions of raving people who have been taken in. Let's say you hear about a new cancer drug. Or your doctor recommends it. So you decide to cover your bases and do your homework first. After looking into it, you conclude it's fine, because all the available information supports its safety and efficacy. But here's what you didn't realize:

- Facebook and Twitter pages promoting the drug are run by people on the drug company's payroll
- The Wikipedia page is controlled by an editor hired by the drug company
- The "nonprofit" organization that recommends it was created and funded by the drug company
- The study you found in your online search was funded by the drug company (most studies funded by drug companies "find" what the company wants them to find)
- The scads of articles reporting positive findings parrot information dished out by the drug company's PR department
- The doctors dismissing concerns about side effects are consultants paid by the drug company
- The lecture your doctor attended – where he decided the

drug was safe and effective – was sponsored by the drug company

And our regulatory agencies are often in bed with these very same drug companies. So don't expect a fix there. What's a person to do? Don your detective hat to see the wolf in sheep's clothing Finding the truth is clearly important to your health. But how do you do that when it's so masterfully hidden? Attkisson provides some tips for recognizing the telltale signs of astroturfing. Once you know them, it'll be easier to recognize the wolves among us.

1. A consistent message everywhere, across the board. Case in point: the line "talk to your doctor" is almost always tied to a drug PR message, even if it doesn't look and smell like an ad.

2. Name-calling. Examples: quack, crank, nutty, paranoid, pseudo, conspiracy, lies...

3. Claiming to debunk "myths" that actually aren't myths at all.

4. Attacking people, personalities, and/or organizations, while failing to address the facts in question. It's like putting a bull's-eye on their back and going after them personally or as a group. It's called an "ad hominem" argument – an attack on the person rather than what he or she is saying. It's an error in logic that was identified nearly 2,500 years ago.

5. Demonizing those who expose wrongdoing, rather than exploring what caused their questions or concerns. Questioning those who question the status quo.

Take this case from 2015:

The American Council for Science and Health (ACSH), a pro-GMO front group, attacked Dr. Mehmet Oz for reporting on scientific evidence of the hazards of glyphosate (the active ingredient in Roundup). Mainstream media had a heyday attacking Dr. Oz – regurgitating vicious propaganda with no critical thought or research. Slate magazine even suggested that Columbia University should fire him for being a quack. The letter proposing this firing accused Dr. Oz of showing "disdain for science and science-based medicine, and baseless and relentless opposition to genetic engineering of food crops." Among the ten "distinguished physicians" who signed the letter was Dr. Henry I. Miller – a well-known paid shill for the GMO industry who's been guilty of multiple falsifications since then. In reality, the attack on Dr. Oz was not orchestrated by "concerned physicians," but by insiders whose job was to attack anyone who raised questions or concerns that might hurt the company's bottom line.

Despite Wikipedia's brutal attacks, Traditional Chinese Medicine (TCM) has a 5,000-year history behind it. Acupuncture is the most prevalent and well-known form of TCM practiced in American clinics. An estimated 14 million Americans have received acupuncture, and its popularity is still rising. Probably the most powerful reason for that is word of mouth from satisfied patients. There's little risk if you go to a certified acupuncture practitioner who uses sterile single-use needles, which is now standard practice. You may be at greater risk if you have a bleeding disorder, a pacemaker, or are pregnant. It might be worth a try.

Importance of journalling daily

There is a unique therapy that lifts and empowers people who are sick, anxious, stressed, or depressed. According to some experts, it improves their outlook and quality of life. Cancer patients use it as a coping mechanism and a way to stay sane (or at least saner) while they undergo treatment. Therapists often suggest it as a treatment for moodiness, depression, and PTSD. It helps you take control of your life and put things in perspective.

So what is this unique therapy? Keeping a journal. Keeping a daily diary is not just for young people trying to figure out their lives. It's a form of self-expression that can be valuable whatever your age or season of life. It can help you navigate through the bumps and bruises of a world where things don't make sense and things don't go perfectly all the time.

The cancer patients who use it (and their therapists who suggest it) may be on to something. Two-time cancer survivor Barbara Tako says she journals whenever life gets really intense and/or her brain starts spinning out of control. She says she wrote about her anxiety to keep from drowning in it. And you can, too – even if you're not a "writer."

The first all-important step

The first step to keeping a journal is to ditch your preconceived notions about it. There's no right or wrong way to do it. You type it, write it by hand, draw or sketch it, or clip it from magazines. Your journal entry of the day can be a rant... or a bulleted list, or a letter you wrote but decided not to send. It can be an email from a friend, a travel log, or whatever. Let go of the rules, regulations, and boxes, and just let it flow. Your diary is for you, and only for you. It's designed to help you clear your head, make important connections about your dreams and struggles, and more.

Journaling can improve your health

This is all very nice, you may think, but can putting words on a page really have any effect on your health? Turns out it can – and does. Letting it all out on a regular basis helps us process difficult events and compose a cohesive narrative about our experiences. This is especially important for those facing challenging health or life events – including cancer, depression, PTSD, grief, and life's general letdowns... Not surprisingly, those who journal regularly recommend it for everyone – healthy or sick, struggling or not. Journaling engages both your analytical, rational left brain and your touchy-feely, creative right brain.

Boosts T-lymphocytes and more

Journaling has very real health benefits. According to an article by Michael Grothaus in Fast Company, it strengthens your T-lymphocyte immune cells. It's also linked to decreased depression and anxiety, and improvements in mood, social engagement, and quality of friendships.

Dr. James Pennebaker is a psychologist and journaling expert. In his seminal study, participants in the experimental group wrote about "past trauma," expressing their thoughts and feelings about it. They were asked to write down their deepest thoughts and feelings about the most horrible experience of their life. Or about an extremely important emotional issue that affected them and their life. The goal was to explore their deepest emotions and connect those emotions to their key relationships.

In contrast, the control group was instructed to write as objectively and factually as possible about neutral topics (such as how they would describe a room or what their plans were for the day). They were told to write without expressing opinions or emotions. Both groups wrote for 15 minutes a day for four consecutive days. They were also told that if they ran out of things to write, they could go back and repeat a topic, perhaps writing about it a bit differently the second time around. They were allowed to write on different topics each day, or the same topic every day. And they were specifically instructed NOT to worry about grammar, spelling, or sentence structure.

All writing was completely confidential. The researchers conducted multiple assessments before and after each subject's four-day journaling stint. The most striking result was that the people in the experimental (expressive) group went to the doctor far less than those in the control group during the few months following the study. Another profound finding was the boost in lymphocyte production among those in the experimental group. Levels of lymphocytes rose during the six weeks of the study. Increased lymphocyte production is a sign of a healthier immune system, which may be behind the reduction in doctor visits.

Some participants reported that while the writing experience upset them, it was also valuable and meaningful. Quite a number of other researchers have replicated and validated the results. The study was NOT a one-off fluke. The Fast Company article also discusses benefits such as faster wound healing, greater mobility for people with arthritis, and more. In short, it looks like blowing off steam in a diary is powerful medicine.

If you're intrigued by the research and want to give it a try, here are some tips to get you started.

1. Try to get used to using a pen again. Hardly anyone does this today. Maud Purcell, psychotherapist and journaling expert, says that most of his patients intuitively know that writing by hand is better than typing. And research supports their intuition. Writing by hand stimulates an area of the brain called the reticular activating system (RAS), which helps us filter and focus on what we're writing. Writing with pen also keeps us from constantly editing what we've written. Even if pen writing is awkward at first, it gets easier with time. Just give it a few weeks.

2. It's for you, not for anyone else. So play by your rules. If you can't stand writing by hand, find the alternative that's best for you. Maybe it's a touch screen, maybe a keyboard.

3. Stick to a time limit. That might mean five minutes, or fifteen. Don't force yourself to fill a certain number of pages. Set a timer and let that be your guide. Then write continuously. Let it flow.

4. There's no "right" time or place to make your daily journal entry. Some people like doing it first thing in the morning, others right before bed. Find a routine that works for you. Journaling in the same place every day can be helpful, but isn't mandatory. Cancer survivor Barbara Tako reminds us that "habits are things that help us, and rules are things that restrict us." Make your decisions accordingly.

5. Don't try to be Shakespeare. This isn't a performance for others to critique. It's for you! Shakespeare wrote for a living, and was a careful observer of human nature for decades. Good for him. But be true to yourself. Stop trying to imitate great writers, and forget about spelling, grammar, sentence structure, and edits. If you're worrying about all those things, you may miss the very point of journaling.

6. Incorporate gratitude into your journaling. Use your journal as an opportunity to reflect (and record) the good things in your life, and to be thankful for them. Gratitude helps reduce symptoms of depression, enables you to reach your goals, and improves social engagement. Plus it boosts long-term wellbeing, reduces pain, and improves sleep. Can you think of even one

downside to gratitude? I can't.

7. Keep it private and secure. Unless you're working with a psychologist who asks you to keep a journal so you can discuss your thoughts at appointments, keep yours private and in a secure place.

If you're going to benefit from journaling, you have to feel free to express things you wouldn't even tell your best friend or your spouse. It has to be a judgment-free zone. Writing a book is for others. Journaling is for yourself. If anything you write could harm your relationships or your reputation, destroy it or put it under lock and key. Journaling is a great habit – whether or not you're suffering (or have suffered) from disease or trauma. It's time well spent.

Regular journaling promotes creativity and propels you toward your goals. It helps relieve stress. Gives you an outlet for your emotions. Facilitates learning through its record of lessons and ideas. Increases gratitude. It provides a reason to push through difficult seasons of life. It's hard to find a downside to this simple habit that only costs a pen and a cheap journal. And its positive effects on your health and wellbeing could be beyond measure.

Flavonoids galore

There's no debate that eating fruit and vegetables is essential to health. In fact, an estimated 7.8 million premature deaths occurred worldwide in 2013 from fruit and vegetable intakes below 800 grams (28 ounces) a day. One of the reasons fruit and vegetables provide such critical nutrition is the flavonoids they contain. Flavonoids are a group of highly diverse compounds -- one of the main subclasses of dietary polyphenols -- found in plants.

The plant produces them to protect itself from pathogens, fungal parasites, herbivores, and ultraviolet radiation. Flavonoids also give color and aroma to plants, which attract insects and birds for the purpose of pollination. So far, around 10,000 flavonoids have been recorded. And they're found in plants that go beyond what we see as traditional fruits and vegetables. Based on each flavonoid's chemical structure, they've been categorized into six main subclasses:

Flavonols - Quercetin, Kaempferol, Myricetin, Isorhamnetin

found in onions, scallions, kale, broccoli, apples, berries, cherries, fennel, sorrel, teas.

Flavan-3-ols - Catechin, Epicatechin, Epigallocatechin 3-gallate (EGCG, abundant in green tea), Proanthocyanidins, Theaflavins found in teas, red wine, cocoa-based products, grapes, berries, apples.

Flavanones - Hesperetin, Naringenin, Eriodictyol found in citrus fruit, fruit juices and prunes.

Flavones - Apigenin, Luteolin, Baicalein, Chrysin found in parsley, thyme, celery, hot peppers.

Anthocyanins - Cyanidin, Delphinidin, Malvidin, Pelargonidin, Peonidin, Petunidin found in red, blue, and purple berries, red and purple grapes, cherries, red wine.

Isoflavones (phytoestrogens) - Daidzein, Genistein, Glycitein found in soyabeans,

You may already be taking some of them as supplements. The health benefits of these flavonoids are vast and boost every part of the body. Chemists summed them up as having: "...antioxidant, cytotoxic, anticancer, antiviral, antibacterial, anti-inflammatory, antiallergic, antithrombotic, cardioprotective, hepatoprotective, neuroprotective, antimalarial, antileishmanial [a tropical parasite], antitrypanosomal [African sleeping sickness] and antiamoebial [pathogenic amoeba] properties."

36 percent fewer cancer deaths

Dr. Nicola Bondonno from Edith Cowan University, Perth, Australia, led an international team of 13 scientists to investigate the link between cancer deaths and the total amount of flavonoids in the diet, as well as the six subclasses of flavonoids considered separately. To do this they looked at data from 56,048 men and women aged between 52 and 60 who had participated in the Danish Diet, Cancer and Health study. They also examined deaths from cardiovascular disease and deaths from any cause (all-cause mortality).

At the start of the study, information about the

participants' diet, education, income, body mass index, smoking status, and alcohol intake, were all taken into account. The researchers also considered risk factors for heart disease and any drugs the participants were taking for heart conditions. They were followed for 23 years, during which there were 14,083 deaths; 6,299 of them were from cancer. The findings, published in Nature Communications in August, showed the more flavonoids in the diet, the lower the death rate from cancer, heart disease and from all causes.

Best protective dose different for cancer and heart disease

The protective effect against heart disease and other causes peaked at 500 mg of flavonoids a day. Beyond this level there wasn't any added benefit. Except when it came to cancer: For cancer-related mortality specifically, the threshold doubled to approximately 1000 mg per day. Dividing the participants' intake into five quintiles, those in the bottom 20 percent of daily flavonoid consumption (173 mg) suffered 1,607 cancer deaths. There were 300 fewer deaths in the next quintile (320 mg daily consumption) with 1,348 deaths, then 100 fewer deaths in the middle quintile (494 mg daily consumption) with 1,240 deaths, and 200 fewer deaths in the next quintile (726 mg daily consumption) with 1,083 deaths. Finally, in the top 20 percent – the people who took the most flavonoids, with an intake at 1,201 mg a day – deaths fell by another 600 to 1,021.

To sum up, the death rate from cancer plunged 36 percent in the quintile consuming the highest daily amount of flavonoids versus the quintile with the lowest daily consumption of flavonoids. The average of 1,201 milligrams taken daily by the high-consuming group is very modest. This is not heavy supplementation at all. It's two or three typical supplement capsules. Another interesting finding: When it comes to flavonoids, variety is a good thing. Each flavonoid subclass is protective This was also the first study of its kind to show each subclass of flavonoid delivers benefits.

After adjusting their findings to take note of dietary and lifestyle factors, the authors observed, "That the thresholds for each of the flavonoid subclasses approximately sum to the threshold for total flavonoid intake is consistent with the idea that all are important and afford added benefit." Commenting on their findings, Dr. Bondonno said,"These findings are important as they highlight the potential to prevent cancer and heart disease by encouraging the consumption of flavonoid-rich foods. "It's important to consume a variety of different flavonoid compounds found in different plant-based food and drink. "This is easily achievable through the diet. One cup of tea, one apple, one orange, 100 grams of blueberries and 100 grams of broccoli would provide a wide range of flavonoid compounds and over 500 mg of total flavonoids." (100 grams is about 3 ½ ounces.) The main source of flavonoids in the Danish population they studied were tea, wine, apples, pears and chocolate.

Smokers and drinkers benefit most

The study found that people at greater risk of heart disease and cancer – smokers and heavy drinkers – benefited most from having a higher flavonoid intake. The added benefit occurs because "flavonoids may protect against some of the detrimental effects that these factors have on nitric oxide bioavailability, endothelial function, blood pressure, inflammation, blood lipids, platelet function, and/or thrombosis, " the researchers wrote.

Yet in obese people, who are also at a higher risk for many of the same reasons, increased flavonoid consumption was only weakly linked to lower mortality. The researchers couldn't come up with a definite explanation for this. However, they suspect the gut microbiome plays a key role because it's known to influence the metabolism of flavonoids and therefore affect their bioavailability to cells. In other words, because obese people have a detrimental imbalance in the ratios of good and bad bacteria in the intestines, they are unable to absorb or use flavonoids in the way people of a healthy weight can.

Acts against most tumor types

Although the study didn't look at the impact of flavonoids on particular types of cancer, other studies have. One study entitled "Flavonoids And Cancer Prevention: A Review Of The Evidence" found flavonoids acted against oral and pharyngeal, gastric, pancreatic, colorectal, liver, prostate, ovarian, endometrial, breast, and lung cancers. A more recent analysis of all relevant population studies from January 2008 to March 2019 also concluded that dietary flavonoid intake is associated with a reduced risk of many forms of cancer. Their review suggested that certain flavonoids are more protective against different types of cancer than others. For example, catechins and flavonols protect against prostate cancer, epicatechin protects against breast cancer, proanthocyanidins protect against lung cancer, and flavones protect against colorectal cancer.

Laboratory research reveals important clues as to why flavonoids might be effective in preventing cancer or stopping its progression. This research shows flavonoids have growth inhibitory effects on various cancer cell types. They act on a number of molecular targets to stop inflammation, cancer cell proliferation, invasion and metastasis, as well as to activate apoptosis (cancer cell suicide).

Eat a variety of flavonoids

These trials focused on individual flavonoids, not the whole group used together. Scientists like to know whether a specific flavonoid is active against the disease, preferring to study quercetin from the flavonols subcategory, or EGCG from green tea for example, rather than look at the whole group of flavonoids used together. It's a basic premise in the science of nutrition that the whole is greater than the sum of its parts, so we need to do as Dr. Bondonno advises in the conclusion of his research: Enjoy a variety of plant-based foods and beverages to gain their full anti-cancer benefits.

Anti-cancer cruciferous foods

And at or near the top of the list is a food often recommended for its anti-cancer benefits: Broccoli. Research proves that it bolsters your cancer defenses by making the anti-cancer genes in your cells more dependable. When a certain food – or ANY outside influence – changes the way genes work, the effect is described as "epigenetic." Genes often need an environmental influence to activate them.

New evidence for broccoli's anti-cancer epigenetic benefits has been uncovered at the Beth Israel Deaconess Medical Center, a teaching hospital for Harvard Medical School. In their tests, the Boston scientists focused on a gene called PTEN – a genetic element well-known for making proteins that suppress tumors. In the body, though, things can run off the track with PTEN. Sometimes this gene can mutate into a warped, dysfunctional form, other times it gets deleted, and still other times it may be inadvertently down-regulated (held back from doing its job properly) – and that's not a complete list of what can go wrong. But when PTEN isn't operating at full capacity, a natural compound in broccoli can give the gene a swift activating kick in the molecular pants.

Broccoli's role in keeping PTEN in working order involves another gene called WWP1. WWP1 can manufacture an enzyme that disables PTEN's ability to hold back tumors. But a chemical in broccoli called indole-3-carbinol can take care of that problem by blocking the production of this troublesome enzyme. "We found a new important player that drives a pathway critical to the development of cancer, an enzyme that can be inhibited with a natural compound found in broccoli and other cruciferous vegetables (like cabbage, Brussels sprouts and cauliflower)," says researcher Pier Paolo Pandolfi.

Get that gene to work

Broccoli's genetic benefits don't stop with blocking this enzyme and the genes that manufacture it. According to scientists at the Linus Pauling Institute at Oregon State University, the sulforaphane contained in broccoli and other cruciferous vegetables can hold back cancer through other epigenetic pathways. Broccoli is a multifaceted cancer fighter – medicine on a dinner plate.

For quite a while, it's been evident that sulforaphane is one of the most important natural, health-giving substances in broccoli. Scientists suspected that this compound played a role in influencing the cellular behavior of enzymes called histone deacetylases (HDACs). HDACs can get in the way of genes that terminate cancer developments in the body.

The Oregon researchers point out that sulforaphane not only inhibits the activity of HDACs, it also plays a role in an epigenetic mechanism known as DNA methylation in a way that reduces the risk of cancer. DNA methylation is a common cellular process that switches genes on and off. In this way, certain DNA material expresses itself and takes part in directing the manufacture of proteins. Other parts of the genetic code are silenced and have to sit on the sidelines without playing a part.

Cellular partners that fight cancer

"It appears that DNA methylation and HDAC inhibition, both of which can be influenced by sulforaphane, work in concert with each other to maintain proper cell function," explains researcher Emily Ho. "They sort of work as partners and talk to each other." Dr. Ho points out that sulforaphane's "one-two punch" moderates this twin pair of genetic activities in the cells and keeps cell division under control. Because when cell reproduction slips its moorings, cells can multiply wildly and form tumors. "Cancer is very complex and it's usually not just one thing that has gone wrong," Dr. Ho explains. "It's increasingly clear that sulforaphane is a real multi-tasker. The more we find out about it, the more benefits it appears to have."

When a cell becomes cancerous, the orderly regulation of gene silencing and activation goes awry. (These functions can also become jumbled in certain types of heart disease, immune system problems and neurodegenerative conditions). "With these processes, the key is balance," says Dr. Ho. "DNA methylation is a natural process, and when properly controlled is helpful. But when the balance gets mixed up it can cause havoc, and that's where some of these critical nutrients are involved. They help restore the balance."

The Oregon researchers also believe that further work on how the compounds in broccoli affect epigenetics involved in cancer could eventually offer an alternative treatment for cancer that isn't nearly as dangerous as chemotherapy. In this vein, other Oregon studies have analyzed how sulforaphane affects what are called non-coding RNAs (IncRNAs). These substances were once believed to be "junk DNA" that did not play an important part boosting cell survival.

Now, researchers have realized that instead of being "junk," IncRNAs play a crucial part in helping genes function correctly. Here, too, when things get out of balance, cancer and other diseases can rage out of control. Research on IncRNA shows that one type in particular, called LINC01116, can lead to cancer when it is dangerously "upregulated" – stimulating cells to reproduce rapidly and spread. "We showed that treatment with sulforaphane could normalize the levels of this lncRNA," says researcher Laura Beaver. "This may relate to more than just cancer prevention. It would be of significant value if we could develop methods to greatly slow the progress of cancer, help keep it from becoming invasive."

The Oregon research demonstrates that when prostate cancer cells encounter sulforaphane, they undergo a four-fold decrease in their ability to colonize and form tumors, because the activity of LINC01116 is restrained. The researchers explain that this same IncRNA is found at high levels in lung, colon and brain cancer. And other misbehaving IncRNAs are present in leukemia as well as stomach, breast and lung cancer.

With all this emerging research on broccoli, it's pretty obvious that anyone concerned about cancer should be eating this and other cruciferous vegetables frequently. To get the biggest dose of the cancer-preventing natural compounds in these foods, eat them raw or very lightly cooked. But no matter how you prepare them, they're going to do good things for your health.

Spicy, hot and dangerous to cancer, that is

Are you a fan of hot spicy food that makes your mouth feel like it's on fire? Personally, I love hot foods every once in a while - I love me some tacos and burritos. Scientists are finding that hot spices are especially suited to fight cancer. Capsaicin -- the natural compound in those foods that burns your tongue -- also turns the heat up on cancer cells and helps keep them from spreading.

It's a natural wonder, and here's how it works. Capsaicin is the ingredient that makes hot chili peppers hot, and at the same time it offers a dream list of exactly the things you would look for if you were searching for a natural substance that can cut off cancer at the knees...

• Blocks genes that help cancer survive.

• Arrests the growth of tumors.

• Stops the extra blood supply that cancer latches onto for nutrients.

• Stymies the metastatic spread of cancer throughout the body.

Persuading cancer to kill itself

Capsaicin often induces cancer cells to commit self-induced suicide, a process called apoptosis that I've often discussed in these pages. The interesting part of capsaicin's role in this process is that it can attack cancer cells in several different ways. Each one of them has the same cancer-destroying result. For instance, it can go after cancer cells' mitochondria, the little organelles that supply the cells with the energy to survive. According to researchers at the University of Maryland, because mitochondria are so central to cancer cell survival – a cell without mitochondria would be like an automobile without an engine – the mitochondria are the "gatekeepers" of the apoptosis process.

So when capsaicin throws a monkey wrench into mitochondrial function, cancer cells conk out like cars ready for the junk heap. Added to that, capsaicin can also activate a gene in cancer cells called p53 – a "tumor suppressor." This gene is involved in the formation of proteins that also lead to apoptosis in cancer cells.

Keep cancer from traveling

Another important trait of capsaicin is its ability to keep cancer from traveling around the body and invading other organs. Most people who die of cancer do so because of this process – called metastasis. It's not the cancer in the original site that kills them. When cancer metastasizes, it becomes more resistant to treatment. That's a big reason metastatic cancer accounts for about four out of five cancer deaths.

Prostate cancer and other cancers commonly metastasize to secondary locations like bone, making these difficult to treat. The natural compound capsaicin from chili peppers could represent a novel therapy to combat metastasis in cancer patients. Capsaicin's ability to disable and kill cancer cells has also drawn a great deal of attention from researchers. Capsaicin has been shown to induce apoptosis.

Researchers at the University of Pittsburgh School of Medicine say the spice helps direct oxidative damage to mitochondria in cancer cells that makes them self-destruct. Plus, other researchers are demonstrating that when capsaicin is combined with other "bioactive food components," the therapeutic effect on cancers is upped considerably. For example a study at the University of Bordeaux in France shows that a combination of capsaicin and resveratrol – an antioxidant found in wine, peanuts, grapes and blueberries – can keep cancer cells from being able to repair damage to their DNA.

When this repair mechanism bogs down, cancer cells are less likely to reproduce and they become more vulnerable to the damage that takes place during radiation therapy – the professional word for this is "radio-sensitized." Likewise, they also become easier to kill with chemotherapy. Not everyone likes spicy foods. But capsaicin is not popular with cancer cells, either. So try some spicy foods. Even if its just adding some paprika when making your omelette, but as discussed earlier, go easy on the eggs to limit arachidonic acid intake.

Organic food - to buy or not?

People often ask if buying organic food is worth the extra money it costs. My usual answer is, "It's worth it if you don't want to eat poison. I don't want to eat pesticides and herbicides." Now there's an exciting extra reason for insisting on organic foods: They contain much higher amounts of cancer-fighting compounds than you'll find in conventional foods.

They provide your organs and immune system with an extra helping of biological weapons they can use to kill off cancer cells. The main reason organic fruits and vegetables provide more anti-cancer protection is the higher doses of natural chemicals these plants make to protect themselves against insects, competing plants and microbes.

A great many species of plants contain such chemicals – for example, one might have a compound that kills or repels insects that try to eat it, another might produce an "antibiotic" to protect against a bacterial pest. An organically grown plant just happens to have higher levels than does the same species of plant grown with the help of chemicals. It's not hard to see why. Conventionally grown crops that farmers treat with pesticides, herbicides and other chemicals don't have to fight for themselves. Organic plants have to produce their own defenses.

Conventionally-grown plants, thanks to a farmer's help, can get by with a less rigorous natural set of self-produced safeguards. In effect, they become lazy, or you could say their "muscles" become weak and their "weapons become rusty." So the studies indicate organic crops manufacture higher levels of those safeguarding substances, and it turns out the same substances can help kill another type of pest: cancer cells. All you have to do is eat them, and they can help your body prevent tumors.

Carrots and celery as cancer medicine

Consider the case of polyacetylenes – a prime example of beneficial cancer-fighting compounds that are more abundant in organic carrots and celery than in vegetables grown with pesticides. Although researchers don't know for sure why carrots and other vegetables make polyacetylenes, their theory is that the substances chase away insects and, when released into the ground, keep other plants from germinating nearby. And research shows that stressed plants that are not treated with pesticides or herbicides make more of these chemicals.

In our bodies, digesting and metabolizing polyacetylenes produces impressive effects that have caught the attention of researchers around the world:

• A study in Denmark shows that polyacetylenes can help muscle tissue fight off oxidative stress that could otherwise damage cellular membranes.

• Research in England shows that polyacetylenes can help kill leukemia cells and keep these cells from reproducing.

• Lab tests show that polyacetylenes can help influence the growth of beneficial probiotic bacteria in the digestive tract that protect against colon cancer.

Full of flavonoids

A class of chemicals called flavonoids is also found in higher levels in organic food. For example, two important flavonoids, quercetin and kaempferol, have been shown to limit inflammation6 and lower cancer risk7. They are found in much higher levels in organic tomatoes than in conventional tomatoes according to tests at the University of California-Davis. The California scientists believe that the fact that organic vegetables are fertilized with manure and compost increases these nutrients. Plus, the slower growth of organic produce may also encourage the extra development of beneficial flavonoids.

Other research demonstrates that flavonoids can:

• Help cells in the body manufacture specialized enzymes that lower the risk of tumors.

• Prevent the harmful oxidation and mutation of DNA.

• Lower the risk of prostate, colon and breast cancer.

Organic meat and dairy

When it comes to picking out meat and dairy, you're also better off with organic. According to a study that involved researchers from a wide variety of countries, cows that eat a 100% organic grass and legume-based diet provide both meat and milk that is richer in omega-3 fats and conjugated linoleic acid (CLA) – nutrients that are good for your health in many ways.

In lab tests, CLA has been shown to stop the growth of cancer cells and keep breast, colon and prostate cancers from spreading and metastasizing. And in a relatively small "proof of principle" study at Dartmouth, researchers found that CLA can disrupt the cell growth of breast cancer by slowing the cells' metabolism of fatty acids. And organic meat's extra omega-3 fats may also may help the body fight cancer. Research at the University of Illinois demonstrates that when your body takes in omega-3s, it manufactures natural chemicals that interrupt the growth and penetration of tumors.

According to the Illinois scientists, our cells use omega-3s to form anti-cancer substances called endocannabinoids – which have some molecular similarities to substances in marijuana but don't produce mind-bending effects. In research, the cancer cells were slowed in their efforts to grow the new blood cells they need for accessing nutrients. The cancer cells also were less able to move around the body and invade other organs, and were more likely to succumb to apoptosis – programmed cell death. The researchers say they were particularly impressed with endocannabinoids' ability to keep cancer cells from migrating into other organs. "The major cause of death from cancer is driven by the spread of tumor cells, which requires migration of cells," says researcher Timothy Fan. "As such, therapies that have the potential to impede cell migration also could be useful for slowing down or inhibiting metastases."

About those pesticides

As mentioned earlier, when you eat organic food you also slash your exposure to pesticide residues in your meals – and many of those pesticides, which are not supposed to be applied to certified organic crops, have been linked to an increased risk of cancer. Now, because pesticides are so widely used and have been previously dumped on farm fields that are now growing organic crops, no matter how much organic food you eat you can't entirely avoid these chemicals. They're too widespread, and some unknown amount of pesticide is often blown onto organic crops from conventional farm fields nearby.

But research in England shows that "the frequency of occurrence of pesticide residues was found to be four times higher in conventional crops, which also contained significantly higher concentrations of the toxic metal cadmium (which is picked up by crops from the soil)." All this research makes it clear why you must eat organic food whenever you can, but without obsessing about it when it's not available. There are clear benefits to eating organic. But if you still eat mostly conventionally produced food, remember that eating plenty of fruits of vegetables is still the most important way you can improve your diet and health, organic or not. Just avoid the "dirty dozen" where possible.

Surprise cancer treatment

Melatonin, sometime referred to as the 'hormone of darkness,' produces physiological changes that help induce sleep, such as reducing body temperature and breathing rate. Melatonin is derived from the amino acid L-tryptophan and is produced within the brain's pineal gland at night. But its role goes well beyond this. Melatonin is not only a hormone but a cell protector that's produced all over the body, impacting almost every cell. Interestingly, the gastrointestinal tract produces more than 500 times as much melatonin as the pineal gland.

Melatonin plays multiple roles in the immune system and has powerful antioxidant and anti-inflammatory properties. Because it can dissolve in both lipids (fats) and water, melatonin easily crosses cell membranes and can even traverse the blood-brain barrier. Through these actions and abilities it protects brain cells from damage, improves cognitive function, combats brain injury trauma including stroke, prevents damage to the heart muscle, speeds wound healing, and reduces pain. But melatonin's most important talent may be the prevention and treatment of cancer.

The role of melatonin in cancer has been thoroughly evaluated, with over 2,000 scientific papers published during the last half century. Scientists have proposed multiple means by which melatonin interferes with the growth of experimental tumors in lab studies. A dozen processes have been put forward, and another dozen potential mechanisms have been suggested.

A research group from the University of Texas, writing in the International Journal of Molecular Sciences in 2017, found it "perplexing" that one compound can act in so many ways to restrain cancer development. They suggested such a diverse range of actions may actually be secondary to a more fundamental process that has yet to be identified.

Here's a brief list of some of the key mechanisms by which melatonin acts against cancer:

1) Strong free radical scavenger. This helps protect DNA from damage and mutation and thereby prevents cancer from getting started in the first place. It also promotes the expression of antioxidant enzymes and reduces the activation of pro-oxidant enzymes.

2) Acts as a pro-oxidant. Like vitamin C, which is an antioxidant at low levels and a pro-oxidant at high levels, melatonin can generate free radicals to directly kill tumors.

3) Limits the cellular uptake of linoleic acid. This omega 6 fat gets converted into a molecule that promotes the proliferation of cancer. This is of particular interest these days, because the standard American diet contains far higher volumes of omega 6 fat than our ancestors ate.

4) Inhibits the activity of telomerase in cancer cells. Telomeres are fragments of DNA that protect the ends of chromosomes. In healthy cells, they become shorter each time a cell divides until the cell is no longer able to divide -- and growth stops. Cancer cells avoid this process of natural cell death by producing the enzyme telomerase, which repairs telomeres and enables cancer cells to keep dividing without limit.

5) Regulates body levels of growth hormone. This is a

critical hormone in cancer development.

6) Prevents angiogenesis (growth of new blood vessels unique to the tumor). Endothelin-1 is a vasoconstrictor secreted by endothelial cells to regulate cell proliferation. It is often elevated in cancer patients. Melatonin markedly inhibits this factor to prevent tumor blood vessel growth.

7) Promotes apoptosis (cell death). Endothelin-1 protects cancer cells from undergoing apoptosis. By inhibiting endothelin, melatonin helps promote the "suicide" of cancer cells.

8) Inhibits metastasis. Melatonin is able to deter molecular processes that help cancer cells enter the vascular system and establish secondary growths at distant sites.

Prostate cancer is more common in middle older age groups, who suffer from declining melatonin levels, and cancer risk is likewise higher in people who are repeatedly exposed to light at night (such as those who work the night shift). In so many studies, researchers found positive evidence for the anti-cancer action of melatonin.

Melatonin not only reduces the toxicity of conventional drugs and increases their effectiveness, but remarkably, it makes cancers that are resistant to treatment with radiotherapy and chemotherapy become sensitive to those treatments. Scientists don't know the reason for this, but they think it's related to the fact that cancer cells have poorly functioning circadian rhythms or clocks and melatonin might help stabilize them.

University of Texas scientists were perplexed about the amazing versatility of melatonin. I should add that they also raised a question: Why isn't it used in regular cancer therapy? They found the evidence "overwhelmingly convincing" for its use, especially as it "lacks any notable toxicity or negative side effects at virtually any dose." Remember, it's inexpensive and non-patentable, so there are no financial gains to be reaped from its use. The Texas team laments that the National Institutes of Health minimally support studies even when many demonstrate substantial cancer inhibition.

Doubles survival

A review of human studies carried out by researchers at the University of Copenhagen, Denmark in 2015 found that melatonin, when used with chemotherapy, increased survival and reduced toxicity in every case. They wrote, "Melatonin significantly improves complete and partial remission as well as the one-year survival rate by around 50%." Joint author Mogens Claesson said, "It seems that melatonin may be an inexpensive and very effective cancer treatment."

Last year, a research group from China published its findings after analyzing 20 randomized controlled trials. Participants in the trials suffered from a variety of metastatic solid tumors, i.e. advanced cancer. The Chinese researchers found the combination of chemotherapy and melatonin doubled the remission rate to 15.57%, compared to 7.07% for chemo alone. The figures for overall survival likewise doubled, 28.24% versus 14.19%. The duration of most trials was one year and patients usually took a 20 mg pill at night. (That's a much larger dose than one would use as a sleep aid.)

Their conclusion was that melatonin "can effectively improve the remission rate and overall survival rate of tumor patients while reducing the incidence rate of neurotoxicity, thrombocytopenia [low blood platelet count] and asthenia [lack of energy] during chemotherapy."

One doctor who has been championing the use of melatonin for some years is Frank Shallenberger, MD, a pioneer and leader in the field of integrative medicine based in Carson City, Nevada. He suggests patients with cancer should take high doses as the "safety data on melatonin is astounding." According to Dr. Shallenberger, nobody has ever discovered a toxic dose. He reveals, surprisingly, that many leading melatonin researchers take 100 mg a day themselves for preventative purposes and that he routinely prescribes anything from 60 to 200 mg a day for his own cancer patients. These seem like staggeringly high doses considering no more than three mg is usually taken to induce sleep – and often much less. The highest dose used in published human cancer trials was 20 mg.

When scientists first tested the effects of vitamin C, they used 100 mg. They thought this was high because it was ten times the amount needed to prevent scurvy. We now know 100 mg is a very small dose. Perhaps melatonin is in the same category. This is supported by a review carried out by scientists in Denmark in 2016. They wrote: "In general, animal and human studies documented that short-term use of melatonin is safe, even in extreme doses. Only mild adverse effects, such as dizziness, headache, nausea and sleepiness have been reported. No studies have indicated that exogenous melatonin should induce any serious adverse effects. "Similarly, randomized clinical studies indicate that long-term melatonin treatment causes only mild adverse effects comparable to placebo."

In spite of the safety data, nobody should be taking melatonin in the kind of doses Dr. Shallenberger suggests. Work with an integrative doctor who can monitor blood chemistry to get the right dose of melatonin. I have typically taken 5-HTP, a processing step ahead of tryptophan to help me sleep while skipping melatonin. Both melatonin and 5-HTP increase serotonin and help with sleep which is detoxifying all by itself. This might be another reason why melatonin helps with cancer.

Herbal treatment for malaria kills cancer too

In the chapter on homeopathy, I brought up a remedy that was similar too the one discussed here - wormwood. This remedy is extremely powerful in treating cancer. Best known as one of the ingredients in the highly alcoholic distilled philosopher's spirit, absinthe, this bushy herb is also found in the cocktail staple, vermouth. Germans call vermouth wermut, which reveals the name of one of the herbs it contains. Wermut translates as wormwood.

Besides being an alcohol additive, wormwood's use as a medicine goes back to ancient times, when it was prescribed for anal pain, to alleviate fever, relieve gastrointestinal problems and later to induce labor and expel parasitic worms -- hence its name. One particular species of wormwood also has considerable anti-cancer properties.

Tames inflammation and helps autoimmune disorders

Wormwood is a member of the genus Artemisia, which

consists of 180 species. The most common type found in the US is Artemisia absinthium. You often see it in flower gardens. Although it doesn't have a flower, it has beautiful silvery-gray foliage. Another variety, Artemisia annua or sweet wormwood, is indigenous to China where it's been used as a treatment for malaria for 2000 years.

Nearly half a century ago, the anti-malarial compound in the plant was isolated; it's called artemisinin. This, along with various drug derivatives (artesunate and artemether are the most widely used), collectively called artemisinins, are now considered a first line treatment for malaria worldwide.

Treats multiple health conditions

Besides its use as an anti-malaria drug, the genus has many other medicinal benefits. Artemisia absinthium has a high content of nutrients and phytochemicals with antioxidant activity. These play important roles in protecting cells and organs from oxidative stress. In a rodent study, an aqueous extract reduced the nerve damage caused by lead poisoning. A similar study, this time with drug-induced liver damage, found that when given beforehand the herb protected the liver. When given afterwards, it restricted the amount of liver damage.

Scientists at the University of Freiburg, Germany, tested Artemisia absinthium in ten patients with Crohn's disease, with another ten acting as a control group. After six weeks, blood levels of TNF-alpha, a pro-inflammatory cytokine, fell from 24.5 to 8.0 in the wormwood group. Among the controls it only fell from 25.7 to 21.1. Clinically, the condition of the disease as measured by the Crohn's Disease Activity Index fell from 275 to below 175 in the herbal group. Among the placebo users, the scores fell from 282 to 230. Remission of symptoms was seen in eight patients in the former compared to only two in the latter.

Artemisinins also possess immunosuppressive properties and are experimentally used to treat autoimmune diseases such as Systemic Lupus Erythematosus, multiple sclerosis, allergic airway disorders, and rheumatoid arthritis in mouse models. In 2017 Artemisia absinthium was tested in a double-blind study in the form of an ointment in patients suffering from osteoarthritis of the knee. The results were compared to patients using a non-steroid anti-inflammatory drug, piroxicam, in the form of a topical gel.

While the drug performed better in relieving joint stiffness, pain relieving effects and improvements in physical function were the same for both groups. Artemisia absinthium also has substantial antimicrobial properties – which makes sense if the genus has activity against malaria -- and has been shown to inhibit the growth of yeast.

Acts like a Trojan horse

The anticancer properties of artemisinins were demonstrated by scientists from the Chinese Academy of Sciences in 1992. Tested against human leukemia, liver, and gastric cancer cell lines, the inhibition rate varied from 82 to 100%. Three years later Henry Lai and Narendra Singh from the University of Washington showed that artemisinin becomes toxic to cancer cells in the presence of iron.

They came up with the idea of teaming the herb with the metal because this is the mechanism by which artemisinin cures malaria. The malaria parasite has a high iron concentration. When the herb comes into contact with the metal it provokes a chemical reaction unleashing a storm of free radicals which attack the parasite's cell membranes, breaking them apart to cause its death.

Iron influx is also high in cancer cells. They need much greater levels to facilitate rapid cell division for tumor growth. It's a general property of all cancer cells. As in malaria, artemisinin becomes extremely toxic, forming free radicals in the presence of iron to kill the cancer cells or cause them to commit suicide. The way it works is that transferrin, the protein that takes up iron, is transported into cells from the blood via transferrin receptors on the cell's surface. The iron-hungry tumor cells take up the transferrin without detecting the attached artemisinin which is bound with transferrin at a molecular level.

Dr Lai explains it this way: "We call it a Trojan horse because the cancer cell recognizes transferrin as a natural, harmless protein. So the cell picks up the compound without knowing that a bomb – artemisinin – is hidden inside." In several studies they found leukemia cells were killed in just eight hours and 98% of breast cancer cells were killed in 16 hours with little harm to healthy cells.

In a later study published in 2008, Lai, Singh and colleagues developed an improved method of delivering iron to cancer cells. Tomikazu Sasaki, chemistry professor at the University of Washington and one of the authors of the study, said, "The compound is like a special agent planting a bomb inside the cell." Unlike toxic chemotherapy that destroys one healthy cell for every ten cancer cells, their new compound kills 12,000 cancer cells for every healthy cell. That makes it an extremely powerful drug with minimal side effects.

Kills many cancers in many ways

An article published in August, 2018 reviewed a large number of studies that had investigated artemisinins. The authors concluded that these herbal extracts have "considerable anticancer properties" aside from the iron mechanism. The herb's other actions include inhibiting proliferation, promoting apoptosis (natural cell death), inducing cell cycle arrest, disrupting cancer invasion and metastasis, preventing angiogenesis (growth of blood supply to the tumor), disrupting cancer cell signaling, and regulating the tumor microenvironment.

The review only covered the previous five years, yet even in that time 150 papers had been published on the herbal compound's anti-tumor properties. Cancer cells that were selectively killed were listed as leukemia, brain glioma, liver, gastric, breast, lung, colon, B cell lymphoma, cervical, head and neck, gall bladder, nasopharyngeal (a rare head and neck cancer), osteosarcoma (bone), esophageal, rhabdomyosarcoma (muscles/soft tissue), schwannoma cells (nerve sheath), pancreatic, ovarian, melanoma, and prostate. "Moreover", they write, "artemisinins have no cross resistance with traditional therapeutic drugs, and they can reverse the multi-drug resistance of tumor cells."

Case reports

In spite of these impressive findings and having an excellent safety profile, being well tolerated and affordable, there's only a scant record of the use of artemisinins in humans. A case report was presented by Dr. Singh concerning a man with cancer of the larynx. After being treated with artesunate for two months, the tumor was reduced by 70%. The treatment was reported to have reduced suffering and prolonged his life.

In a personal communication to California integrative physician Robert Rowen in 2002, Dr. Singh said he was following a number of cancer patients and there was "nearly universal improvement on artemisinin or its derivatives." Dr. Rowen himself also reported a number of successes. One example was a case of Non-Hodgkin's lymphoma which showed up as an egg-sized tumor on the side of the head. It spontaneously cleared up just four weeks after a course of artesunate.

Dr. Len Saputo, another integrative physician practicing in California, likewise claims many successes. One of these was a woman in her sixties with advanced lymphoma that had spread to large parts of her body. He reported that she was alive, asymptomatic and doing well four years into taking the herbal extract.

Human trials

Dermatologists in Germany experimented with artesunate "on a compassionate use basis" for two metastatic melanoma patients, as an adjunct treatment to chemotherapy. One experienced a temporary response, while the other saw stabilization of the disease and regression of metastasis. He was still alive 47 months later even though the average survival time for this condition is two to five months.

A randomized, double blind, placebo-controlled pilot study was published in 2015. Researchers at St. George's, University of London gave 22 patients with colorectal cancer either oral artesunate or placebo. 42 months following surgery there were six recurrences of cancer in the placebo group (out of 12 patients) but just one out of ten among those taking artesunate. Survival beyond two years in the artesunate group was estimated at 91% while surviving the first recurrence of cancer in the placebo group was only 57%.

Professor Sanjeev Krishna, who jointly led the study, said, "The results have been more than encouraging and can offer hopes of finding effective treatment options that are cheaper in the future." The other lead author, professor Devinder Kumar, a leading expert in colorectal cancer at St George's, added: "Larger clinical studies with artesunate that aim to provide well tolerated and convenient anticancer regimens should be implemented with urgency, and may provide an intervention where none is currently available, as well as synergistic benefits with current treatment regimens."

How to take artemisinin

Artemisinin is available as a supplement. The dosage recommended with active cancer is between 200 mg and 500 mg per day. The derivatives are only available through a physician. And it appears most of the studies have been on the derivatives. After five to seven days, absorption of artemisinin in the digestive tract falls substantially, so advocates of this treatment recommend it be taken for four consecutive days, followed by three days where none is taken. This cycle can then be repeated.

In less than one percent of cases it can cause inflammation of the liver. This does no permanent damage but the supplement would have to be stopped. There may also be concerns with people who have too much or too little iron in their bodies. Such people should proceed cautiously.

The homeopathic remedy I discussed earlier in the book may be far better with little or no side effects. I urge you to revisit the chapter on homeopathy and go with that treatment if you have side effects from the supplement.

Send in the stem cells

There is a natural way to increase healthy stem cells that have been depleted by cancer treatment. This way to increase stem cells is with a cocktail of L-carnosine, green tea and blueberries. Studies show that this cocktail spurs the growth of stem cells. The combination is also very healthy.

Other studies of blueberries show this fruit can prevent and even reverse cell functions that decline as a result of normal aging.29-36 Blueberry extract has been shown to increase neurogenesis in the aged rat brain. Green tea compounds have been shown to inhibit the growth of tumor cells, while possibly providing protection against normal cellular aging. Based on these findings, scientists are now speculating that certain nutrients could play important roles in maintaining the healthy renewal of replacement stem cells in the brain, blood, and other tissues. It may be possible, according to these scientists, to use certain nutrient combinations in the treatment of conditions that warrant stem cell replacement.

A common side effect of cancer chemotherapy drugs is bone marrow damage, leading to immune suppression and other blood disorders. Medical oncologists routinely prescribe expensive drugs such as granulocyte-macrophage colony-stimulating factor (GM-CSF)—which is also naturally produced by the bone marrow—to stimulate bone marrow stem cell activity. These drug treatments are not without risks of side effects.

When combinations of nutrients were tested, however, a greater percentage of bone marrow cell proliferation occurred compared to GM-CSF. For example, a combination of blueberry and vitamin D3 exhibited a 62% increase in proliferation of bone marrow cells. Blueberry and catechin (green tea extract) increased bone marrow cell proliferation by 70%. When carnosine and blueberry were combined, the growth promotion observed was 83% . . . an effect significantly greater than that of the expensive drug GM-CSF!

The scientists next tested various nutrients on early stem cells, which can be identified and isolated by their surface antigen-receptor expressions (e.g., CD34 + and CD 133 +). The GM-CSF drug increased these early stem cells by 48%, as expected. A combination of blueberry, green tea, vitamin D3, and carnosine, however, increased these stem cells by an astounding 68%. So go for the trio, you may be pleasantly surprised by the benefits.

The power of spirituality

A famous celebrity cancer survivor is quick to credit the overwhelming support from fans. "I've got a couple million people out there who have expressed their good thoughts, their positive energy directed towards me and their prayers," he said. He believes his healing is due to more than the chemo. His doctors would agree.

Can science explain the human spirit?

The simple truth is that prayer is becoming more widely acknowledged as a way to cope with cancer. But what does that process look like? And why does it work? Hundreds of researchers over the past two decades have performed various studies as they try to answer these questions. The goal is to get a better picture of how this mysterious healing element plays out in the body – and how it can be consistently replicated.

Even the NIH, which refused before the year 2000 to consider research proposals with the word prayer, has since funded multiple studies on the topic. We're now seeing systematic investigations and clinical research into the world of spirituality, complete with professional societies that publicly support this effort.

Consider a pilot study managed by Mitchell Krucoff, MD, a cardiovascular specialist at Duke University School of Medicine. His group looked at the effects of "distant prayer" on patients who undergo high-risk procedures like angioplasty. The outcome of Dr. Krucoff's study was that distant prayer did not have a measureable effect on the primary clinical outcome of heart procedures, but it did seem to prompt therapeutic effects such as relief of emotional distress, plus lower re-hospitalization and death rates.

Dr. Krucoff's 2005 study, published in The Lancet, was the first time rigorous scientific protocols were applied to prayer. Combined with the results of similar studies, it gives us useful insight into how technology-laden health care intersects with the role of the human spirit.

Call it what you want: It works

Of course, what prayer means to one person may be entirely different to the next. The Buddhist and Hindu form of prayer is meditation. For Catholics, the Rosary is a favorite. Some Protestants practice centering prayer, which places a strong emphasis on interior silence. And there are certainly other forms of prayer.

What all types of prayer have in common is a physical effect on the brain. MRI scans reveal complex brain activity occurs as an individual goes deeper and deeper into concentration. The frontal and temporal lobe circuits, which track time and create self-awareness, disengage during deep prayer sessions, and the limbic system becomes more active.

This is key, because the limbic system regulates your heart rate, blood pressure, metabolism, and nervous system. The limbic system is sometimes called the "premammalian" part of the brain because it is found in lower orders of animals. It's "pre-cognitive," if you will.

Once a person has achieved a meditative state, what happens is fascinating. As scientists describe it, the awe and quiet people feel during prayer or meditation takes place because everything starts to register as emotionally significant. As your body relaxes during a prayerful session, physiological activity gets more evenly regulated.

Some consider the experience a connection with God. The materialist just thinks it's the result of brain activity. Either way, prayer and meditation have tangible effects on health. Scientists explain it as inducing a worldview that gives you more perspective on problems and makes it easier to get through ups and downs. And because of that, you're more likely to be optimistic and hopeful about recovery from disease and less likely to experience as much stress as a non-religious, non-prayerful person might endure.

When others step in for you

The brain activity of a prayerful person makes sense if that person is doing her own praying. But how do you explain the benefits of distant prayer, like the celebrity above experienced with his fans?

This type of prayer-for-others is called intercessory prayer, although some have now dubbed it "prayer therapy." The goal is to accomplish some form of healing – though healing means different things in different situations.

Still, the general hypothesis behind intercessory prayer is that it motivates a spiritual force or energy that accomplishes healing in some way, whether that means helping people suffer less pain or stress, get out of the hospital faster, require less medicine, or similar positive effects.

In 2017, actor Val Kilmer attributed prayers and good thoughts from around the world for his healing from throat cancer, along with his Christian Scientist faith and chemotherapy.

Without it, high-tech medicine falters

As the saying goes, "God helps those who help themselves." There's a fantastic array of effective treatments available for cancer and many other diseases. We would be foolish not to take advantage of them while we pray or meditate (which we should be doing when healthy, anyway.)

Still, it's possible that high-tech medicine missed the boat. In its pursuit of all things machine- and technology-driven, Western medicine has done a bang-up job of ignoring the rest of our human needs. And as it turns out, by giving prayer and positive thought a seat at the table, it's likely all that high-tech stuff will work better overall.

At any rate, whether or not our current version of scientific studies can prove it, prayer continues to be a significant source of solace and strength for individuals going through a crisis. Its benefits are clearly measurable today.

Newly discovered organ may play a role

It seems incredible that scientists have discovered a new human organ. How did they miss it so far? Well, they did. A new organ has been identified. Actually, two. Plus a new "structure" that is not quite an organ.

First, the "structure": In 2017, an elaborate system of drainage vessels was seen in the brain for the first time. Until then their existence was suspected, but not certain. And then there's the mesentery. Thought to be just a few fragmented structures in the digestive system, the mesentery was found to be a single structure and has now been officially reclassified as an organ.

But the third and last is the most important: Last year another suspected new organ was discovered called the interstitium. It may be a big factor in cancer. Remarkably, if confirmed, the interstitium will become the largest organ in the human body by volume. This previously unseen structure may change our understanding of many body processes affecting both health and disease, and the reason some forms of alternative medicine work the way they do. It might also explain how cancer spreads throughout the body.

A fluid-filled three-dimensional latticework

Dr. Neil Theise, a distinguished pathologist at Mount Sinai Beth Israel Medical Center, New York, and New York University School of Medicine, went to work on a routine day, several years ago. Two of his colleagues, David Carr-Locke and Petros Benias, part of an interdisciplinary research team, approached him with an unusual image they'd seen with the help of a new instrument called a probe-based confocal laser endomicroscope. This device allows scientists to view living tissue in detail within the body.

To study what they'd seen under a microscope, tissue samples were removed from the patient, quick frozen, cut into thin slices and amplified with a green dye, so differences in microscopic structures could be seen clearly. Viewing the large duct that drains bile from the liver, they could see dark bands separating a strangely shaped, bright, fluid-filled three-dimensional latticework of proteins, connective tissue (bundles of collagen and elastin) and unknown cells. No one had ever seen this phenomenon before.

In further research, scientists uncovered the mysterious latticework everywhere they looked. Under the skin; lining the gastro-intestinal tract, urinary system and lungs; in the fascia between muscles; and in connective tissue surrounding arteries and veins. The structure makes up one-fifth of all fluids in the body - a huge 10 liters.

A pre-lymphatic highway

To Dr. Carr-Locke "it became clear that this was a

previously unrecognized universal system throughout the body that connected certain organs with each other." The three scientists together with eight other colleagues published their findings in Scientific Reports last year. Whether this can be classified as a new organ, as they suggest, will have to be confirmed by other research groups.

Although their existence was known, these fluid-filled spaces – making up the interstitium (from the Latin meaning the space between) -- had never been seen because, under normal circumstances, tissue samples are fixed in formalin before they're observed under a microscope.

Formalin is a solution of formaldehyde, which kills living cells. Its use clears the fluid from the interstitium sample and collapses the spaces so they appear solid on biopsy slides. This caused the scientist on the other end of a conventional microscope to assume he was just looking at a dense wall of collagen alone. Sometimes faint little white cracks could be seen in it, but these were thought to be tears in the tissue. Now they know these are remnants of former interstitial spaces.

The researchers described the interstitium as a pre-lymphatic highway of moving fluid that drains into the lymphatic system and ends up in the lymph nodes. The lymphatic system is an extensive network of vessels that helps rid the body of waste and transports fluid containing white blood cells -- lymph -- throughout the body.

The researchers believe the interstitium serves as a shock absorber for tissues because it can be compressed, stretched and expanded, and is seen in all moving parts of the body. They also think it plays a role in edema – an unhealthy condition in which excess fluid accumulates in body tissues. But the effects of the interstitium could be more far reaching.

A potentially important diagnostic tool

Commenting on the implications of their discovery, Dr.

Theise said, "If this organ is present in every tissue and other organ the way the cardiovascular and lymphatic systems are, then we have an incomplete understanding of the entire body. "This is basic anatomy, basic physiology. I don't think there's anything that doesn't get changed by this." For example, he suggests that maybe fibromyalgia has been such a medical mystery "because we haven't recognized the compartment of the body that's affected."

Dr. Michael Nathanson, head of digestive diseases at Yale University School of Medicine, agrees that the New York team seems to have uncovered "a completely new concept" which could become altered in disease or play a role in driving disease. Dr. Theise and colleagues think that as the cells and collagen bundles in the interstitium change with the aging process, they may contribute to skin wrinkling, limb stiffening, and the progression of fibrotic, sclerotic and inflammatory diseases.

Although the cells in the interstitium cannot be identified as yet, the scientists believe they could be mesenchymal (adult) stem cells, which can contribute to the formation of scar tissue seen in inflammatory diseases. Dr. Theise added that their findings have the "potential to drive dramatic advances in medicine, including the possibility that the direct sampling of interstitial fluid may become a powerful diagnostic tool."

Increases understanding of alternative medicine

Surprisingly for an orthodox scientist, he said the protein bundles seen in the space are likely to generate electrical current as they bend with the movements of organs and muscles around them, and may play a role in techniques like acupuncture. In an interview he added, "And this is where people who are interested in fascia, such as osteopaths or some people who do body work like Rolfing or cranial-sacral practices have been saying, that fascia also has fluid. "But allopathic trained doctors like me and conservative anatomists of the world say, 'No, when you look at it under the microscope, fascia is just dense connective tissue. What do you mean there's fluid there? There's no fluid there.' "

Dr. Theise said one of his hopes from publishing this paper is that the osteopathic community would now have an anatomic explanation for their practices. As you can see, Dr. Theise is no ordinary pathologist. For the last 30 years he's practiced Zen Buddhism and yoga, and has given talks on theories regarding acupuncture and the seven chakra points, and how yogic practices influence cellular and molecular biology.

The cancer link

As part of their research, the New York scientists examined tissue from five patients with cancer of the stomach and skin (melanoma) to see if cancer cells were present in the interstitium. And that's exactly what they found. If cancers are able to invade the interstitium and extend into the lymph nodes, this could explain how tumors spread, especially those in the GI tract, they believe. "This makes perfect sense when you consider the classic pattern of bile duct metastases," Dr. Carr-Locke explained. "This tissue plane of the interstitium is very loose, which would make it easy for the cancer to spread up and down the duct before spreading outward."

If this is a first step to how cancer spreads, it could lead to new ways of preventing it. Dr. Carr-Locke continued, "It certainly would have implications for how we treat a tumor surgically. "We know that manipulating a cancer can often spread cells from exposed surfaces; you can often see metastatic disease occur fairly soon after a tumor is resected. Maybe that happens through the interstitium, and maybe targeting that is an important step in oncology."

Professor James Williams at the Department of Cell & Molecular Medicine, Rush University in Chicago, agrees that the interstitium likely plays a key role in spreading cancers of the GI tract and possibly other cancers, and could change the way doctors treat cancer and other diseases. The presence of the interstitium clearly shows how alternative cancer therapies such as acupressure and osteopathy can work whose effects were hitherto unknown to Western medicine.

And in the same way why exercise is clearly beneficial to fighting cancer as we discussed earlier as it facilitates movement that activates the interstitium. Another excellent reason to move daily! The same would explain the therapeutic benefits of massage which also help cancer patients find some much needed relief during treatment.

Combine integrative and conventional medicine

Not enough people take advantage of the "best of both worlds," alternative and conventional. Some doctors today advocate marrying conventional and natural medicine instead of choosing an either-or protocol... because they feel there can be great synergy between the two.

This is especially true for aggressive cancers, where time is of the essence. Synergistic strategies support your mitochondria – the tiny "batteries" inside your cells – thereby enhancing your immune system while countering the side effects of conventional therapies. After all, the stronger your normal cells are, the less likely they'll get recruited to be cancer cells.

Dr. Paul Anderson is a naturopathic doctor practicing in Seattle, Washington. He also practices at a clinic in Rosarito, Mexico – where they're able to use therapies they can't use in the

U.S. He has practiced integrative oncology for more than 20 of the total of 42 years he's been a doctor. He stumbled into oncology when patients began asking him about cancer.

He recently co-wrote a book on integrative oncology with Dr. Mark Stengler, another naturopathic medical doctor, in which they describe the various integrative protocols and combinations they employ. Dr. Andersen is adamant that "if diet's not your first and last strategy, you'll never beat cancer."

Fighting an aggressive cancer demands a ketogenic, low-carb environment. By this he means a strictly monitored clinical ketogenic diet – not merely the basic lifestyle/fitness keto diet that is widely popular. In his view, patients should have a Ketone meter and closely monitor their ketosis levels under the care of a medical professional. If cancer is less aggressive or in remission, he recommends you start with fasting, and follow with a whole-food, raw vegetable diet that includes juicing. Then settle into a Mediterranean diet for the long term.

Naturally everything in this protocol should be as clean as possible – organic, GMO-free and pesticide-free. There's no point in flooding your body with more carcinogens to fight. To sum up, the dietary protocol is keto, coupled with intermittent fasting, plenty of fiber, and MCTs (medium chain triglycerides). And lots and lots of clean filtered water.

This is the beginning and the end, the alpha and the omega, he says. Without it, no other treatment will work. It's even more true when a sneaky, late-stage cancer appears suddenly, out of the blue.There are many people who had no idea they were sick, then learned that, inside, they were riddled with metastatic cancer.

But he says the eating recommendations also hold true when a patient is told that all signs of cancer are gone. That's when patients often make the mistake of changing back to their pre-cancer habits. They stop doing the very thing that worked so well in their favor.

Dr. Andersen also recommends other supplements to help enhance your mitochondrial function, keep cells from being recruited as cancer cells, and support your body through the treatment process.

CoQ10 - This nutrient can help address defects in energy metabolism and oxidative damage that play a role in the pathology of brain diseases.

High-dose IV curcumin - The IV form of this turmeric extract is not yet widely available (and obviously requires a doctor), but taking curcumin by mouth can help. Curcumin mitigates the negative effects of chemo and radiation, sensitizes your cells to conventional therapies, and helps protect your healthy cells.

Vitamin C - Contrary to what oncologists have believed for decades, vitamin C turns out to be synergistic with chemotherapy – as studies have demonstrated.

Boswellia - Fights pain and inflammation, helps repair genes, supports the immune system, prevents infections, and more.

Vitamins K2/D3 - This potent anti-tumor agent inhibits cancer cells, induces apoptosis (natural cell death), and more. Vitamin D3 inhibits proliferation and stimulates differentiation. These two vitamins should be taken together.

Take your next step today

Dr. Andersen believes survival boils down to diet, ketone esters, hyperbaric oxygen, and glutamate control. As stated above, he also advocates conventional treatments, especially in the case of aggressive late-stage cancers where quick action is needed. These supplemental natural treatments assault cancer cells, protect stem cells and keep them quiet, and help the immune system recognize cancer cells so they can no longer evade detection.

Dr. Andersen mission is to help people clean up their diet, create a lifestyle that supports wellness, and incorporate a supplement regimen that gives every possible chance for other treatments to work. And also to make sure you're not left in a position where your body is so beat up that cancer can return with a vengeance.

This protocol can also act as a stand-alone treatment for those who are so advanced in years or in such an advanced stage of cancer that it would kill them to undergo conventional treatment. But never say never - because people have recovered from the worst of circumstances. While you don't have to follow what Dr Anderson says(I did not), the important point is to keep an open mind. It may just save your life.

Fear and psychology of cancer

Some people die of something else and their cancer is only discovered by chance post mortem. Some people just fight back with a fury and they win!

Cancer is feared too much. This fear is played upon by oncologists, who want your money. Some of them try to hoax you that if you don't start their treatment within a week, you're a goner anyway. The truth is cancer is not erased by killing off tumors--that's given rise to the myth that it will come back. It will come back because the root cause disease has not been addressed.

Cancer is gotten rid of by eliminating the causes. Treating the end-result (the tumor) is a fool's game. That includes, by the way, treatments that are just substitutes for chemo, like laetrile, DCA and Protocol. Those treatments are toxins (laetrile is basically cyanide) and what I call "chemo-mentality". None of these substances have a place in the healthy human body.

There are a very few REAL treatments for cancer. In fact there are just four ways to truly conquer cancer:

1. Diet and nutrition
2. Chemical clean-up
3. Improving oxygenation of the cell tissues
4. And one other very important and often forgotten element in fighting cancer:

The psychology of battling cancer is absolutely CRUCIAL. We know the mind is powerful. It can heal by its own intention. Keep that in mind daily.

Epilogue

It was another dreary and rainy day in November 2018 when I stepped out of my car and into the vast offices of my urologist in Dallas. The urologist had one look at my case history(I was coming to see him after almost 9 months) and was surprised to see me. He asked why I had returned. I told him I was undertaking active surveillance and wanted him to check if I had stayed the same or regressed since our visit(of course I knew better and was secretly hoping he would see an improvement but I wanted to know how much). The nurse had my PSA test and the urologist proceeded to give me a prostate exam.

He gave me a funny look soon after. Curious and feigning fake concern, I asked him what he had found. He said he had found nothing! Not even the smallest iota of prostate lumps, hardness or enlargements, it was all gone!

Happy, I pressed him further. He said the PSA tests had come back and my PSA was now down to 1.2, which was now not only normal but a vast improvement from the 6.5 levels and this had happened in just eight - nine months! Curious he asked me what treatment I had taken and where I had taken it. With a deadbeat look, I told him that I had completely eschewed eggs for the last nine months and that had likely helped.

Now distinctly irritated, and likely guessing I was pulling his leg and would likely offer no more details (I would not), he dismissed with a curt smile and told me to continue doing whatever it is that I had been doing. He would not need to see me again unless I reported similar issues again in the future. Happily I made my way back to my car to report the good news to my wife. Five years later, I have never returned to that office and my PSA levels continue to stay in the 1.2 - 1.5 range with no symptoms whatsoever.

If there is a lesson here, it is what you too can do what I have done, incredible as it may seem. And what's more, you can do this by yourself not just once or twice, but as many times as you need to. The three prongs help me keep cancer at bay and I expect it will help you too. To you my friend, I say "Live long and prosper!"

CANCER DOES NOT HAVE THE FINAL WORD.

THE END.

References

Flavanoids as AntiCancer Agents, PubMed Central PMC7071196

The role of Vitamin D in cancer prevention, National Library of Medicine Dec 2005

Cancer inhibition by green tea, PubMed PMID:9675322, Jun 1998

Homeopathy in Cancer (HINC) Study protocol Jan 10, 2011 ClinicalTrials.gov

"22 Case Studies Where Phase 2 and Phase 3 Trials had Divergent Results", US Food and Drug Administration, January 2017

Made in the USA
Monee, IL
14 January 2025

76878888R00144